GUT
FEELING

DELICIOUS **LOW FODMAP**
RECIPES to SOOTHE THE
SYMPTOMS of a SENSITIVE
— GUT —

GUT
FEELING

DELICIOUS LOW FODMAP
RECIPES to SOOTHE THE
SYMPTOMS of a SENSITIVE
GUT

LORRAINE MAHER & PAULA MEE

GILL BOOKS

Gill Books

Hume Avenue

Park West

Dublin 12

www.gillbooks.ie

Gill Books is an imprint of M.H. Gill & Co.

© Lorraine Maher and Paula Mee 2017

978 07171 7261 0

Designed by Jane Matthews

Photographed by Joanne Murphy www.joanne-murphy.com

Styled by Orla Neligan of Cornershop Productions www.cornershopproductions.com

Assisted by Jane Flanagan

Edited by Kristin Jensen

Indexed by Adam Pozner

Printed by Replika, India

PROPS

Meadows & Byrne: T: 01 2804554/021 4344100; E: info@meadowsandbyrne.ie; meadowsandbyrne.com

Marks & Spencer: T: 01 2991300; marksandspencer.ie

Article Dublin: T: 01 6799268; E: items@articledublin.com; articledublin.com

Dunnes Stores: T: 1890 253185; dunnesstores.com

Harold's Bazaar: T: 087 7228789

TK Maxx: T: 01 2074798; tkmaxx.ie

Golden Biscotti ceramics: goldenbiscotti.bigcartel.com

The Patio Centre: T: 01 2350714; thepatiocentre.com

Industry Design: T: 01 6139111; industrydesign.ie

Sostrene Grene: sostrenegrene.com

TWI Fabrics Ireland: T: 01 8553777; fabricsireland.com

Flying Tiger Stores: ie.flyingtiger.com

This book is typeset in Fira Sans and Camilla.

5 4 3 2

Note

This book is intended as a reference guide only, not as a medical manual. It is not a substitute for any treatment that may have been prescribed by your doctor. If you suspect you have a gut problem, please seek medical help. Bear in mind that nutritional needs vary from person to person. The information discussed here is intended to help you manage your IBS or IBS-like symptoms and is best used in conjunction with your dietitian or GP.

Acknowledgements

This book would not have happened without the help of our friends and family, especially Sinead Dempsey, Cian O'Dwyer, and Alan, Lilah and Edith Maher. Thank you all. Although there are far too many to mention, we really do appreciate your support. A very special thanks to the great team at Gill Books – including Sarah Liddy, Deirdre Nolan, Catherine Gough, Teresa Daly, Kristin Jensen, Orla Neligan, Joanne Murphy and Jane Matthews – who were ever-present and helpful along the way.

Contents

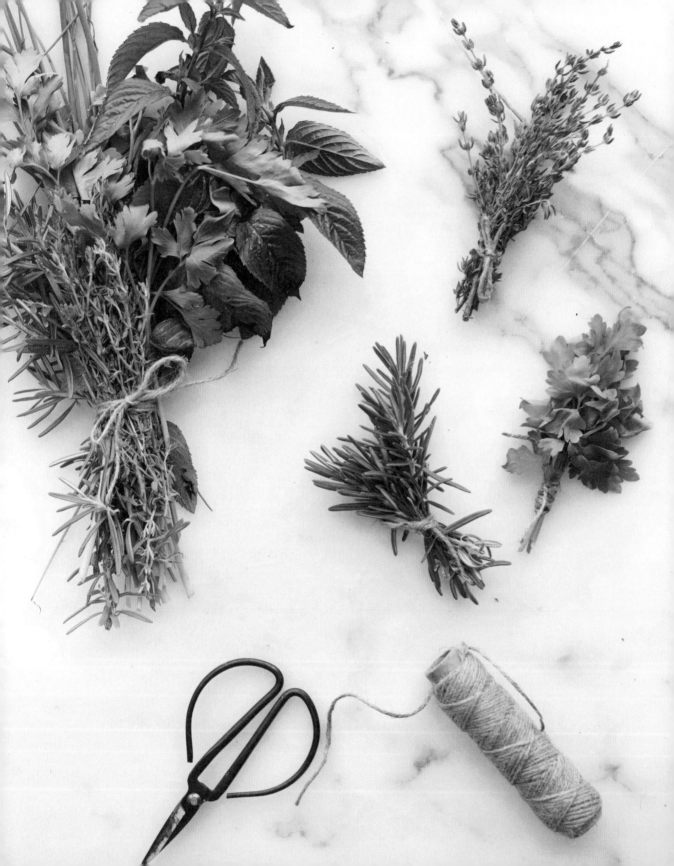

Introduction

As dietitians, we meet patients with digestive conditions such as irritable bowel syndrome (IBS) on a weekly basis. Their lives are often turned upside down by their embarrassing symptoms. Having both undertaken additional training for the low FODMAP diet, our experience in gut health has made work with these patients more valuable and gratifying as we see people's lives return to normal. Distressing symptoms frequently abate and emotional anguish is reduced.

The approach we take with our gut patients has been carefully and vigorously tested by top researchers around the world. More than 30 clinical trials have investigated the new approach known as the low FODMAP diet, and the evidence is so convincing that many national bodies, including the Irish Nutrition and Dietetic Institute (INDI), the British Dietetic Association (BDA) and the National Institute for Health and Care Excellence (NICE), have incorporated it into their evidence-based guidelines for the management of IBS.

Bowel conditions affect as many as one in five people and IBS is particularly common in young women in their 20s and 30s. Some manage and some struggle while getting on with their lives, but many feel wretched if symptoms consistently interfere with their enjoyment of food and their ability to live a normal life.

While IBS is not a life-threatening condition, depression is common in those who have it. Sadly, some severely affected patients have even contemplated suicide. The good news is that research shows that at least 70 per cent of people with IBS find that their symptoms either improve or are resolved following the low FODMAP diet described in this book. (Previous interventions yielded a meagre 30 per cent improvement in symptoms.)

GUT THERAPY

This book provides practical advice and delicious recipes to help you manage gut issues using the principles of the low FODMAP diet. This is an elimination diet that excludes certain carbohydrates known to aggravate gut problems and digestive conditions.

The low FODMAP diet can help more than just those experiencing IBS symptoms. It can improve gut symptoms in more than half of patients with inflammatory bowel diseases (IBD) such as ulcerative colitis and Crohn's disease. In particular, it helps people who have endured ongoing gut symptoms despite having inactive IBD. It is also under review as a potential therapy for gut symptom relief in women with endometriosis and for patients recovering after bowel surgery. It may also be helpful for those who live with other unspecified bowel disorders or SIBO (small intestinal bacterial overgrowth).

Times are changing in the medical world too. The vast majority of gastroenterologists now believe that changes in diet are as effective as, or even better than, taking medications for IBS.

Whatever the issue, this book can help you identify foods that trigger your specific gut symptoms, tailor your cooking skills and recipes and modify your meal plans to omit particular culprit foods in the long term. There are tasty meal suggestions and tips for everyone, whether you're a busy student, a frazzled weight watcher or simply under pressure at work.

Ideally, a dietitian specifically trained in this field should supervise you on the low FODMAP diet. In fact, we specifically designed this book to complement the personalised advice you can get from a dietitian.

 It's important to note that the low FODMAP diet does not cure IBS, ulcerative colitis, Crohn's disease or unspecified bowel disorders. What it *does* offer is real relief and effective management of your symptoms.

Stop the guesswork, get the answers

You might think you know which foods trigger your symptoms. You may have eaten something as part of a meal and then shortly afterwards you began to feel unwell. It's easy to see how foods get labelled as 'no-no' or problem foods. For example, if you ate a stew with chicken, onions, carrots and rice and felt unwell, you may think the rice is the reason why you felt bloated, when in fact the onion is the trigger. We often hear of foods wrongly denounced like this in our clinical practice, but we understand how it can easily happen.

The time a food takes to travel through the gut varies from one person to the next. It can even vary in the same person from day to day. The key thing to note is that the travel time takes hours, not minutes, so blaming a food you have just eaten for your IBS symptoms is not necessarily a good idea. It's more likely that the symptoms were caused by foods you ate much earlier or from a build-up of FODMAPs consumed during the day.

So guesswork is tricky and not recommended. It can result in unnecessary food restriction on the basis of a hunch. When entire food groups are avoided (all dairy, for example), this in turn may lead to a deficiency of a nutrient, e.g. calcium, unless you make up for the lost nutrient. In the longer term, bone disease or osteoporosis may result if the diet remains poorly balanced.

Avoiding certain foods can be perplexing, especially if you tend to focus on all the things you can't eat. Then there are the additional hassles of reading food labels, briefing a waiter when eating out, finding appropriate recipes and eating a wide variety of the food groups that are important for our gut and overall health.

Gut Feeling will help you focus on the impressive list of foods you *can* eat. We provide you with simple and relevant substitutions for the foods you have to remove while following the first stage of the low FODMAP diet plan (which should be followed for a maximum of eight weeks only). The objective is to minimise gut symptoms initially by strictly following the low FODMAP diet and then eventually help you resume and enjoy the most varied and wholesome diet possible.

 The low FODMAP diet is not designed to be a long-term diet. It is a temporary intervention to uncover your personal trigger foods. It is not a cure for bowel disorders, but rather a tool to help you self-manage your symptoms in the long term.

WHAT IS THE LOW FODMAP DIET?
FODMAPs: What are they?

FODMAPs is an acronym for different components of carbohydrates that are difficult to pronounce! It's not necessary to remember their names. FODMAPs are neither 'good' nor 'bad'. They are simply food components that people with gut sensitivities find difficult to digest.

* FODMAPs are found in carbohydrates.
* They are not found in proteins and fats.
* Healthy carbohydrate-rich foods such as apples, garlic and milk contain FODMAPs.
* Not-so-healthy processed carbohydrate-rich foods like battered fish, croissants and biscuits contain FODMAPs too.

Luckily, not all carbohydrate-rich foods are high in FODMAPs. You can still include specific carbohydrates, especially when you really need them during your day. This might be first thing in the morning after an overnight fast or after a training session or activity.

FODMAPs stands for:
* **F**ermentable
* **O**ligosaccharides
* **D**isaccharides
* **M**onosaccharides
* **a**nd
* **P**olyols

Examples of carbohydrate-rich foods containing FODMAPs

FERMENTABLE	FODMAPs are fermented in the gut by bacteria. These bacteria produce hydrogen, methane and carbon dioxide gases, which can distend the tummy area.
OLIGOSACCHARIDES	Fructans found in wheat, rye, onions and garlic. Galacto-oligosaccharides found in legumes and pulses.
DISACCHARIDES	Lactose found in milk, yogurt and cheese, and anything made from these.
MONOSACCHARIDES	Fructose found in honey, apples and mangos.
POLYOLS	Sugar polyols (e.g. sorbitol, mannitol and xylitol) found in sugar-free mints and gum and certain fruits and vegetables.

This book does not provide a complete list of FODMAPs. Lists are continually being reviewed and updated, so beware of misinformation on out-of-date blogs or Facebook pages. A dietitian will provide you with the most up-to-date list as well as any relevant personalised advice. She may also suggest an appropriate app for your smartphone that will help you with recommended portion sizes and allowed foods when grocery shopping so that you don't have to memorise long lists of foods to avoid. In addition, the amount of FODMAPs in carbohydrate-rich foods can vary depending on where the food is grown, the climate and soil fertility. It's not advisable to simply lift information from the internet, as the advice will only be relevant to the country of origin.

 You can download the FoodMaestro Ltd app called FODMAP from the Apple app store. It contains relevant FODMAPs for Ireland and the United Kingdom, including many branded foods.

FODMAPs: What do they do?

We all experience some difficulty digesting FODMAPs. That's normal. However, FODMAPs are a serious problem for the hypersensitive gut. They can cause symptoms in numerous ways.

* They are not effectively digested or absorbed where they should be in the small intestine. This means they continue along the gut, into the large intestine.
* They are osmotic and draw in more water than is necessary into the gut.
* They are fermented by bacteria that produce excessive amounts of gas.

The gut can therefore be swollen or distended by solids (undigested FODMAPs), liquids (excessive water) and gas (produced by bacteria). This can lead to pain, bloating, visible tummy ballooning, excessive wind, diarrhoea or constipation.

The hypersensitive gut picks up these intestinal changes rapidly and communicates with the brain through its nervous system. It seems able to observe and feel pain at a lower threshold compared to a normal gut.

By reducing FODMAPs – hence the name 'the low FODMAP diet' – you can reduce the malabsorptive, osmotic and fermentative side effects, which helps reduce or eliminate gut symptoms in the hypersensitive gut.

What to expect on the low FODMAP diet

There are three stages in the low FODMAP diet. A consultation with a FODMAPs trained dietitian before you start each stage is advisable. If you don't have access to a dietitian, then we recommend that you purchase the FoodMaestro Ltd FODMAP app (see above).

Stage 1: The exclusion stage

At your first consultation, your dietitian will give you a list of foods high in FODMAPs to exclude for a minimum of two weeks and up to eight weeks. Some people report improvements in their symptoms pretty quickly after starting the first stage. For others, it takes the full eight weeks to get relief.

In this book we have included a list of alternative foods you can enjoy instead of some of the high FODMAP foods you will be asked to avoid. You can expect better improvements in your symptoms the closer you stick to the diet. You aren't seeking perfection here, just your very best effort to exclude high FODMAP carbohydrates.

Stress and anxiety can worsen your symptoms, so before you begin, make sure you have the time to plan and give Stage 1 (the exclusion stage) your full commitment. Half-doing it is a waste of your time!

 It's important to realise that this is not a no-FODMAP diet! The exclusion stage is only followed for a period of two to eight weeks, not indefinitely.

What can you still eat? Nutritious carbohydrates such as quinoa, oats, potato and rice are allowed on the low FODMAP diet. There are plenty of suitable vegetables (carrots, green beans, spinach and tomato) and fruit (bananas, passion fruit, oranges and strawberries) to choose from. An increasing number of dairy alternatives are available too (lactose-free milk and soya products). Proteins (lean meat, poultry and seafood), fats (certain nuts, olive and rapeseed oil) and sweet foods like a little dark chocolate are not restricted either.

So what can you use instead? You can see from the swap list on the next page that there are some FODMAP foods that you can eat in very small amounts. For example, you can eat a quarter of an avocado but not more than that, otherwise you may trigger symptoms. And don't forget that the effects of FODMAPs are cumulative. In other words, eating small quantities of several low FODMAP foods at one meal can be just as problematic for the gut as eating a large quantity of a single high FODMAP food.

Although this is not a comprehensive list, these are common foods that you need to avoid, but we list suitable alternatives for when you are preparing or cooking meals. If you focus on the foods in the white column and make a list of the foods you like, you can make a suitable shopping list from the options available. Remember, too, that portion control is important. Where a portion size is specified, eating more than the recommended portion can cause symptoms in some people with IBS.

FODMAP swap list

FODMAPS TO AVOID	LOW FODMAP
Wheat-based cereals	Porridge, cornflakes, Rice Krispies, buckwheat flakes
Wheat-based pasta and noodles	Wheat-free or gluten-free pasta, quinoa, rice, rice noodles, 100% buckwheat noodles, potatoes
Bread (including products such as wraps, pittas and pizza bases)	Gluten-free breads, wheat-free breads, 100% spelt sourdough bread (no honey), taco shells
Couscous, gnocchi	Polenta
Wheat flour	Gluten-free flour, almond flour, corn flour (cornmeal), rice flour
Crackers, biscuits, muffins, pastries, croissants, rye crackers	Rice cakes, corn cakes, oatcakes, gluten-free or wheat-free biscuits, gluten-free or wheat-free cakes, gluten-free or wheat-free pastries
Onion, leek	Radish, ginger, chives, spring onion (green part only), asafoetida powder
Garlic	Garlic-infused oil
Mushrooms	Courgette, aubergine
Savoy cabbage	White cabbage, red cabbage, bok choy, spinach
Cauliflower	Turnip, parsnip
Stewed apple	Stewed rhubarb, stewed raspberries
Watermelon	Honeydew melon, cantaloupe melon
Blackberries	Raspberries, blueberries, strawberries
Nectarines	Clementines, mandarins, oranges
Mango	Pineapple
Milk (including goat and sheep milk, buttermilk, evaporated milk and condensed milk)	Lactose-free milk*, calcium-fortified soya milk*, almond milk*, coconut milk*, rice milk*
Yogurt (in quantities >50g), fromage frais	Lactose-free yogurt *, soya yogurt *

Check ingredients to avoid problem fruit, fructose and inulin

FODMAP swap list

FODMAPS TO AVOID	LOW FODMAP
Cream cheese (in quantities >50g/2 tbsp)	Lactose-free cream cheese
Ricotta, quark, reduced-fat Cheddar, processed cheese	Soft cheese (except extra-light versions), Cheddar, Camembert, goats' cheese, feta, brie, blue cheese, mozzarella, Parmesan
Ice cream	Soya ice cream, sour cream, cream, crème fraîche
Baked beans, dried beans, including lentils, chickpeas, soya beans, black-eyed peas, butter beans, kidney beans and split peas	Eggs, Quorn, firm tofu, canned lentils and chickpeas (<42g)
Breaded meat, battered meat	Beef, pork, lamb, chicken, duck, turkey
Breaded fish, battered fish	Fish (tinned, fresh and frozen), shellfish
Pistachios, cashews	Macadamias, pecans, pine nuts, walnuts, peanuts, Brazil nuts, sesame seeds, sunflower seeds, pumpkin seeds, flaxseeds/linseeds, chia seeds, almonds (<10), hazelnuts (<10)
Blackberry jam	Raspberry jam, strawberry jam, blueberry jam, marmalade
Honey, agave nectar	Maple syrup, golden syrup, sugar
Gravy and stock	Homemade versions, such as the ones in this book
Sugar-free mints, sugar-free chewing gum, sugar-free chocolate	Mints, dark chocolate, white or milk chocolate (<30g)
Apple juice, pear juice, mango juice, dandelion tea, chicory tea, chamomile tea, fennel tea, coconut water	Water, peppermint tea, black tea, green tea, red tea, coffee in moderation, herbal teas, decaffeinated tea, decaffeinated coffee
Very sweet wines, e.g. dessert wines, rum (avoid any drinks that make symptoms worse)	Most alcoholic drinks

Note: Brands may vary, so double-check labels for FODMAP ingredients.

Stage 2: The reintroduction stage

After the two to eight weeks of the exclusion stage, a review appointment with your dietitian is necessary. At this consultation your symptoms and their severity will be re-evaluated. Next, the business of reintroducing specific FODMAP foods is discussed. Reintroductions are done in a particular order. Small amounts of the excluded foods are reintroduced in each three-day period and the dose or amount of the food being tested is increased to find your tolerance level. You will be asked to keep a written record of any symptom that arises as you proceed through these specific food challenges. Your dietitian may provide a small handbook where you can document your results.

Most people enjoy this stage, as it allows them to test certain favourite foods (e.g. onion, garlic and avocado) that they have missed. However, it's important to complete each and every challenge first before you integrate all the tolerated foods back into your diet. Some foods will be reintroduced without causing upset, whereas others will cause a symptom to return, sometimes with a vengeance. You identify your trigger foods at this stage.

Stage 2 can take up to eight weeks depending on how many food challenges you carry out.

Stage 3: The modified diet

At the final consultation, your dietitian will help you compile your IBS management plan for the long term. Many people return to their normal diet with perhaps a few high FODMAP foods to avoid or consume in smaller amounts.

If there are many foods to avoid, a dietitian will ensure you will not be nutritionally compromised following a modified diet in the long term.

Avoid getting information from the internet. It may not be accurate or relevant for you specifically.

Why not cut out carbohydrates completely? Do we need them?

A certain amount of carbohydrate is important for health. Carbohydrates provide us with an energy source for the brain and working muscle. The by-products of carbohydrate digestion (certain fibres) are also essential food for the good bacteria in the gut. Having a healthy microbiome (gut bacteria) is important to support a healthy immune system.

The first stage of the low FODMAP diet restricts many carbohydrate-rich foods. Look at this stage as a timely opportunity to focus on eating unrefined and high-fibre sources of carbohydrates, rather than a license to eat lots of wheat- or gluten-free versions of starchy (bread) or sugary (biscuits, cakes) foods. There is the prospect of building new healthy habits for the long term during this time. Your waistline and your gut will benefit when you reduce unwanted calories from highly refined carbohydrates (see the weight loss advice on pages 197–198).

On the other hand, if you are underweight, we have some suggestions for how you can maintain or gain weight while still following the initial restrictive first phase of the low FODMAP diet (see the weight gain advice on pages 199–200).

We have included the calories per portion and other relevant nutrition information beside each recipe to help steer you.

The low FODMAP diet and fibre intake

Avoiding wheat-based foods and perhaps some of your favourite fruits and vegetables in Stage 1 can reduce your fibre intake substantially unless you're careful. With approximately four out of five adults not eating enough fibre as it is, finding suitable alternative fibre-rich options is particularly important during Stage 1.

Gradually increasing low FODMAP foods, like oats, oat bran and linseeds, will provide a good source of soluble fibre. Oats are commonly taken as porridge, homemade granola or muesli for breakfast, but can also be used as a cooking ingredient, as a topping on fish, crumbles or in oatcakes.

Oats are considered to be a high-fibre food: a 40g serving provides 10 per cent of the guideline daily amount (GDA).

The potential fibre content of a porridge-based breakfast

Food	Fibre
40g oats	2.5g
150ml rice milk	0.8g
1 medium banana, chopped	1.5g
3 walnuts, chopped	1.0g
Total Sufficient fibre-rich foods = 25g/day	**5.8g fibre** 23% GDA

Other fibre-rich allowed foods

You may need to increase or decrease your fibre intake depending on your symptoms (see also pages 206–207).

* **Aubergine:** This low-calorie vegetable is a particularly good source of soluble fibre.
* **Nuts:** During Stage 1, pistachio and cashew nuts are not allowed and almonds and hazelnuts are restricted to fewer than 10 nuts per day. However, all other nuts are allowed and are a great addition to your diet.
* **Seeds:** Linseeds/flaxseeds, chia, sunflower and pumpkin seeds are all nutritious as well as good sources of fibre. If you suffer from constipation, linseeds/flaxseeds may help (up to 2 tablespoons per day for a three-month trial), but be sure to consume them with plenty of fluid (approximately 150ml per tablespoon of seeds). It is also recommended to increase the amount gradually by 1 teaspoon per week to figure out your optimal dose.
* **Grapes, strawberries, kiwi and citrus fruits:** These fruits are rich in pectin, a type of soluble fibre that lowers bad cholesterol and which can have positive effects on the bowel and overall health.
* **Soya mince:** Soya mince is a great vegetarian source of fibre.
* **Fibre supplements:** Supplements offer the least appealing way to get soluble fibre. Two teaspoons a day of psyllium, which is found in some bulk-forming laxatives, provide about 4g soluble fibre. Discuss fibre supplements and laxative use with your doctor.

What about fats and proteins?

Fats and proteins are FODMAP-free. However, the hypersensitive gut will find a lot of fat in one meal difficult to digest. A large fried breakfast is not advised! **What to do:** Focus on healthy fats found in oily fish (salmon, mackerel, tuna and sardines) once or twice a week, use olive or rapeseed oil when cooking and eat a small handful of allowed nuts every day as a snack. (See the list of allowed nuts in the swap list on page 8.)

Some protein at each meal is ideal. Unfortunately, many of the plant proteins (beans, chickpeas and lentils) are predominantly restricted during the first stage of the low FODMAP diet. (See the list of allowed legumes in the swap list on page 8.) **What to do:** Focus on amino acid-rich proteins such as eggs and grilled sardines for breakfast; cheese, tofu and shellfish as lunch options; and all kinds of seafood, poultry, lean beef, lamb and pork at dinner.

While processed meats (such as salami, ham, chorizo and bacon) are very tasty, they are not good for our general health. For this reason, we have made a conscious effort to avoid them in our recipes. We realise that they add lots of flavour, so if you do decide to add some, just use them sparingly and make sure they don't contain FODMAPs.

PLANNING AND SHOPPING

Planning your meals in advance can make a big difference to your ability to stick to the diet. If you know what you will be eating for each meal and have stocked up in advance, you are much more likely to eat the right foods.

* Stock up on plastic containers for freezing meals when you batch cook.
* Plan your meals three days at a time and prep them in advance as much as possible. For example, on Sunday prep food for Monday, Tuesday and Wednesday, then do the same for the rest of the week on Wednesday evening. Cut up allowed veggies in bulk ahead of time and refrigerate them properly in a sealed plastic bag.
* Bag up smoothie ingredients too. By measuring out your berries, lactose-free yogurt (freeze it in an ice cube tray) and greens ahead of time, your smoothie will be perfectly portioned every time and speedy to put together.
* Establish a personal core list of suitable foods for Stage 1 on your supermarket's webpage. This makes weekly shopping easier and you can shop from your bespoke list day or night.

Core shopping list
Fresh foods
* Allowed salad veg (tomatoes, cucumber, beansprouts, chives, endive, rocket, iceberg lettuce, spinach leaves, radishes, red, orange, yellow and green peppers)
* Allowed fresh vegetables for roasting and cooking (aubergines, carrots, courgettes, parsnips, olives, swedes/turnips and yams)
* Allowed fruits (citrus: limes, oranges, lemons; berries: blueberries, strawberries, raspberries; everyday fruits: bananas, grapes, kiwi, rhubarb, honeydew and cantaloupe melons; exotic fruits: papaya, pineapple, passion fruit)
* Lactose-free dairy or suitable rice or soya alternatives (watch out for apple juice sweetener)
* Stick to cheese such as feta, Camembert, Brie, goats' cheese, mozzarella, Edam, Cheddar or a little blue cheese
* Fresh herbs (basil, coriander, parsley, rosemary, thyme, green part of spring onion)
* Poultry (chicken, turkey) and eggs
* Lean cuts of pork, lamb and beef
* All white fish, shellfish and oily fish (salmon, tuna, sardines, trout, mackerel)

Store cupboard essentials

* Brown, wild or basmati rice
* Breakfast cereal, e.g. porridge oats, pinhead oatmeal, oat bran
* Garlic-infused olive or rapeseed oil (for cooking)
* Basil- or chilli-infused oil (extra virgin olive oil, for dressings)
* Dried herbs
* Tinned fish (e.g. salmon, tuna, sardines, mackerel)
* Fish sauce, soya sauce, oyster sauce
* Green tea or red tea (these contain more antioxidants and less caffeine than black tea)
* Spices (e.g. chilli, cinnamon, ginger, mustard seeds, nutmeg, black pepper, turmeric)
* Condiments (e.g. asafoetida powder, mustard, white rice vinegar)
* Seeds (e.g. sesame, sunflower, pumpkin, chia, linseed, poppy)
* Nuts (e.g. peanuts, pine nuts, pecans, walnuts, macadamia nuts)

Frozen foods

* Frozen vegetables (spinach, green beans, carrots)
* Frozen fruit, e.g. berries (except blackberries) – perfect for adding to desserts
* Prawns, crab or fish

TIME TO GET COOKING
Cooking without garlic and onions

The bad news is that both onions and garlic cannot be eaten during Stage 1 of the diet. The good news is that there are umpteen suitable herbs and spices that can add great flavour to food when garlic and onions are restricted. Make sure you have a selection of the following herbs and spices in your kitchen at all times.

* **Garlic-infused oil** is widely available in supermarkets and is FODMAP – and hassle-free. If you want to make your own, cut a few peeled garlic cloves into slices and sauté in oil for 1–2 minutes, until a garlic flavour develops. Then you must fish out and discard every single garlic slice, even the tiniest pieces.
* **Asafoetida powder** (also known as hing) is an interesting Indian spice that you can find in Asian and health food shops. It has a pungent and not very pleasant smell, but when heated in oil it gives it an onion flavour. You only need to use a pinch to get the effect and this works well in curries, soups and stocks.
* **Spring onion, the green part only**. Discard the white parts or throw them on someone else's plate.
* **Chilli**
* **Chives**
* **Fresh herbs** (parsley, thyme, rosemary, basil, coriander)
* **Spices** (cumin, turmeric, coriander, paprika, cinnamon)
* Fresh **lemons** and **limes**
* **Maple syrup**
* **Vinegar** (red or white). You can use balsamic, but not more than 1 tablespoon.
* **Mustard**
* **Peanut butter**
* **Salt** and **freshly ground black pepper**

 Both capsaicin (a compound found in chilli) and menthol (a compound found in mint leaves) act on the same receptor in the mouth, but in different ways. Chilli deceives the body into thinking it's hot when it's not, while mint has the opposite effect. So take a cue from great Asian food and combine minty aromatic herbs in side salads to counteract and complement hot, spicy dishes.

How to use the recipes in this book

The recipes in this book are divided by mealtimes (breakfast, lunch, dinner.) as well as for specific needs. For example, you might want recipes that are lower in calories or higher in fibre, so these symbols were designed to help.

High fibre
for constipation (>6g/serving)

High carb
for endurance sports (4g carbs : 1g protein)

Weight management
Breakfast <300 kcals, light meals <400 kcals,
main meals <500 kcals and snacks <150 kcals

Spicy food
containing chilli (including garam masala
or curry powder) and cayenne pepper

We wish you happier times preparing and enjoying delicious and nourishing family-friendly meals. Here's to getting back on track and embracing life and food again. Good luck!

Note: **A food in bold type** *must be portion controlled. In other words, you can have the amount specified in the recipe, but if you eat more than the recommended serving of the* **food in bold type**, *it can trigger symptoms.*

Small amounts of gluten can be tolerated on a low FODMAP plan except for those who suffer from coeliac disease. To help those who have been diagnosed as coeliac, dishes that contain gluten have been identified in the list of allergens for each recipe.

A note on allergens

We cannot guarantee that every allergen in the recipes will be identified and labelled in the allergen list, as food and condiment manufacturers could change the formulation at any time. If you are concerned about food allergies, you must be aware of this risk and double-check all the ingredients to the best of your ability.

Breakfast & Brunch

We all know the **value** of a good breakfast, but when you're following a new diet it's even more important to have something to eat early in the day so that you are less likely to **snack** on the wrong things mid-morning in a moment of weakness. Mornings can be **hectic** for many of us, so it's handy to have a list of breakfast options that can be prepared in minutes or in some cases eaten **on the go**. For days when you have a bit more time, we've included some great breakfast and brunch recipes that the whole **family** can enjoy.

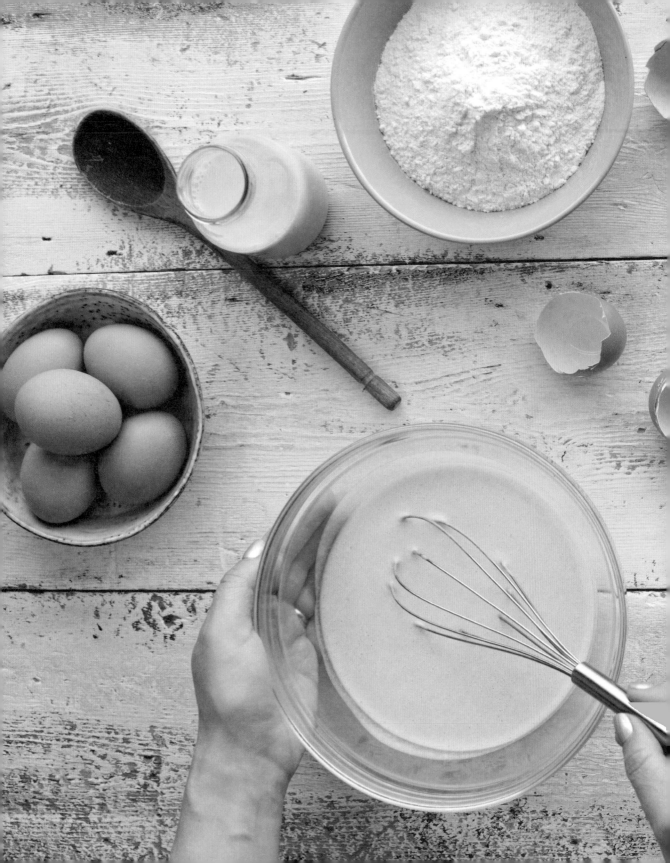

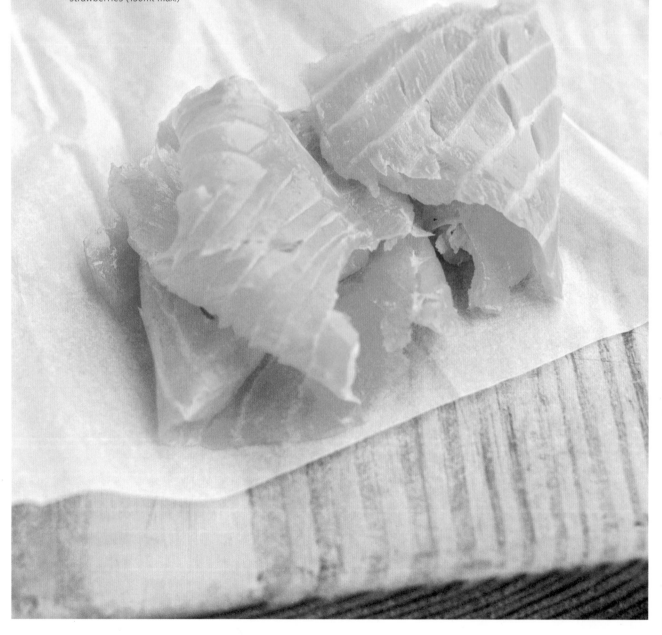

Quick breakfast ideas

* Gluten-free cereal with lactose-free or soya milk and berries
* Gluten-free toast with peanut butter and banana slices
* Gluten-free bagel with smoked salmon, **1 tablespoon low-fat cream cheese** and ¼ avocado
* Scrambled eggs and cherry tomatoes
* Strawberry smoothie blended with lactose-free milk or yogurt and strawberries (150ml max.)

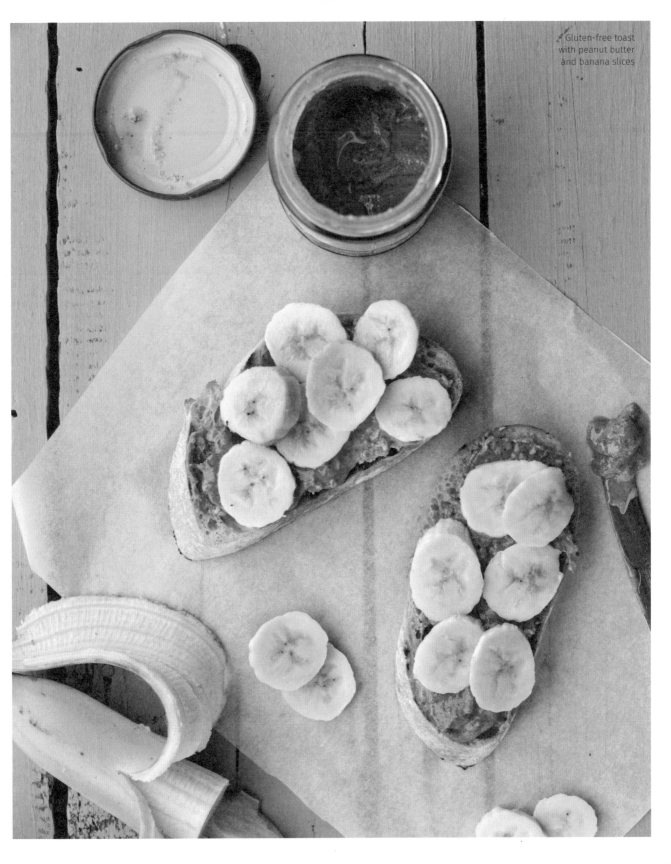

Gluten-free toast
with peanut butter
and banana slices

BREAKFAST

Bircher Muesli

Developed around 1900 by a Swiss doctor, Maximilian Bircher-Benner, for his hospital patients, this breakfast includes a chilled concoction of rolled oats and other grains, fresh and dried fruit, seeds and nuts and may be mixed with plant milks. Nowadays it's known as overnight oats. Favourite toppings include 100g strawberries or the seeds of one passion fruit or 10 crushed almonds. Simply remove the muesli from the fridge and let it stand for a few minutes as you make your morning tea, then enjoy!

  Portion size: 251g **Kcals:** 486 **Fat:** 28g **Saturated fat:** 2.5g **Carbs:** 40g **Sugar:** 16.6g **Fibre:** 11.4g **Protein:** 13.9g **Salt:** 0.02g **Allergens:** Tree nuts, may contain gluten

INGREDIENTS

100g/1 very ripe banana

60g oats

1 dessertspoon sunflower seeds

1 dessertspoon chia seeds

1 dessertspoon linseeds

300ml almond milk

1 tbsp maple syrup

WHAT TO DO

1 Mash the banana in a large bowl, then add the oats, seeds and almond milk. Stir in the maple syrup, then cover the bowl with cling film and leave overnight in the fridge, until it thickens.

2 The following morning, top your bircher muesli with whatever allowed fruit you like.

Preparation time: 10 minutes
Cooking time: N/A
Serves: 2

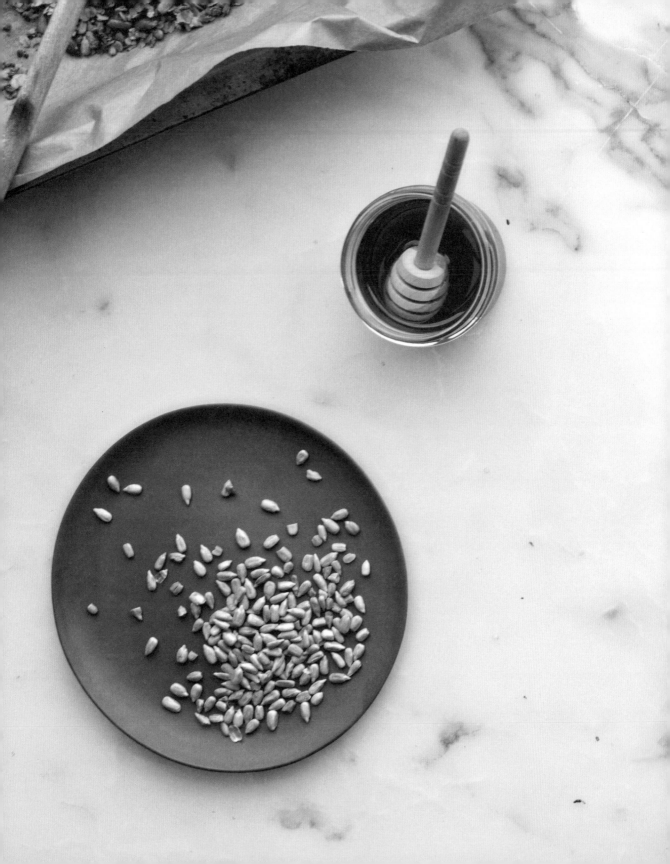

Coconut and Mixed Seed Granola

Serve this crunchy granola with some fresh strawberries or raspberries and a few dollops of natural yogurt. **On the low FODMAP diet you can use up to 50g (max) of natural cow's milk yogurt and up to 18g of desiccated coconut.** It's worth adding these for great taste and texture.

 Portion size: 78g **Kcals:** 374 **Fat:** 23g **Saturated fat:** 6.3g **Carbs:** 29g **Sugar:** 5.2g **Fibre:** 8.9g **Protein:** 8.2g
Salt: 0.01g **Allergens:** Tree nuts, may contain sesame, may contain sulphites, may contain gluten

INGREDIENTS

200g porridge oats

6 tbsp chia seeds

3 tbsp sunflower seeds

2½ tbsp pumpkin seeds

50g desiccated coconut

3 tbsp rapeseed oil

2 tbsp maple syrup

2 tsp vanilla extract

WHAT TO DO

1 Preheat the oven to 180°C.

2 Mix together the oats, seeds and coconut in a large bowl.

3 Heat the oil and maple syrup together in a small pot set over a medium heat, but don't let it boil and burn. Remove from the heat and allow to cool before adding the vanilla.

4 Combine the wet and dry ingredients, then spread the granola out evenly on a baking tray.

5 Bake in the oven for 20–25 minutes, until it's nicely toasted. Allow to cool completely, then store the granola in an airtight container for the week.

Preparation time: 10 minutes
Cooking time: 30 minutes
Serves: 6

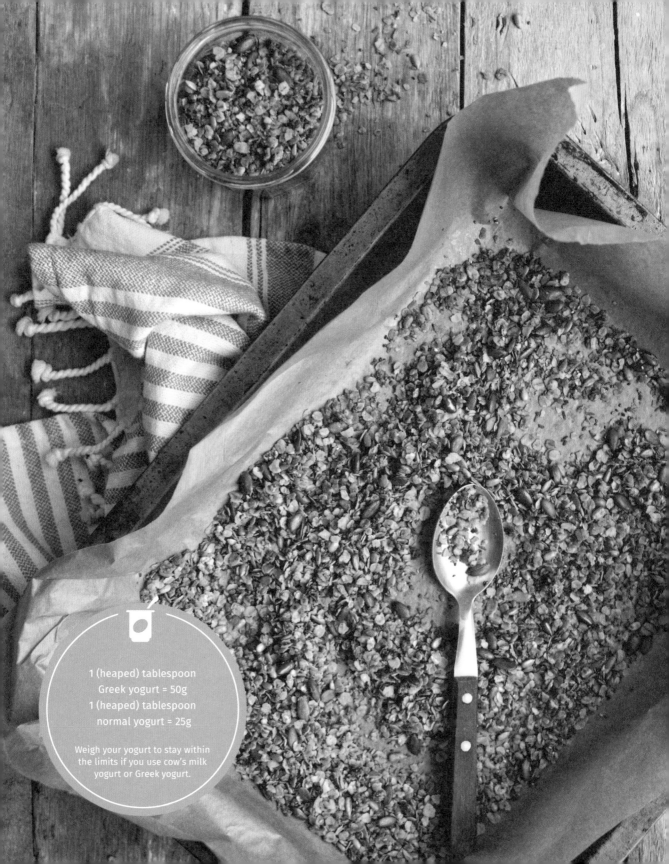

1 (heaped) tablespoon
Greek yogurt = 50g
1 (heaped) tablespoon
normal yogurt = 25g

Weigh your yogurt to stay within
the limits if you use cow's milk
yogurt or Greek yogurt.

Hot Berry Porridge

Wake up and start your day with a warm bowl of berry porridge. It's easy to make and it fuels you for the day ahead. Blueberries are not only deliciously sweet, but they are also packed with antioxidants, which are essential for keeping your body in great running order.

   Portion size: 330g* **Kcals:** 291 **Fat:** 9g **Saturated fat:** 1.1g **Carbs:** 38g **Sugar:** 9.9g **Fibre:** 9g **Protein:** 8.8g **Salt:** 0.01g **Allergens:** Tree nuts, may contain gluten *Analysis is based on using water, not rice milk.*

INGREDIENTS

90g pinhead oatmeal

315ml water or rice milk

1 tsp ground cinnamon

200g blueberries

2 tbsp flaked almonds

1 tbsp linseeds

WHAT TO DO

1 Place the oatmeal and water in a pot and bring to the boil, then reduce the heat and simmer for 5 minutes. Stir in the cinnamon and cook for a further 2 minutes.

2 Divide the porridge between two bowls and stir in the blueberries. Sprinkle the flaked almonds and linseeds over the top and serve straight away.

Preparation time: 5 minutes
Cooking time: 7 minutes
Serves: 2

Quinoa Spinach Scramble

A balanced scrambled egg! It's also a great way to use up leftover quinoa.

  Portion size: 335g **Kcals:** 380 **Fat:** 21g **Saturated fat:** 5.9g **Carbs:** 18.9g **Sugar:** 4.4g **Fibre:** 6.3g
Protein: 24g **Salt:** 1g **Allergens:** Eggs, milk

WHAT TO DO

1 Whisk the eggs with the milk and season generously with black pepper.

2 Heat the oil in a pan set over a high heat. Add the spinach and let it wilt, tossing the leaves continuously, for about 2 minutes. Sprinkle the grated nutmeg on top.

3 Pour the egg mixture into the spinach and let it sit for about 20 seconds before stirring gently with a wooden spoon, lifting any egg off the bottom of the pan.

4 Let it sit for about 20 seconds before stirring again. Repeat until the eggs are soft but still runny, then add the quinoa. Cook for another 1–2 minutes, until heated through and the eggs are set.

5 Spoon onto a plate and serve with grated Parmesan and extra black pepper.

INGREDIENTS

4 eggs

50ml lactose-free milk

freshly ground black pepper

1 tbsp garlic-infused olive oil

200g spinach

1 tsp grated nutmeg

185g cooked quinoa

1½ tbsp grated Parmesan

Preparation time: 10 minutes
Cooking time: 5 minutes
Serves: 2

Exotic Fruit and Yogurt Parfait

A delicious, nutritious and refreshing way to start the day! **Be sure to only take one portion per sitting if using soya coconut yogurt, as the guideline amount is <125g per sitting.**

Portion size: 488g **Kcals:** 252 **Fat:** 3.6g **Saturated fat:** 0.5g **Carbs:** 31g **Sugar:** 30.6g **Fibre:** 9.8g **Protein:** 7.5g **Salt:** 0.3g **Allergens:** Soya

INGREDIENTS

400g/1 papaya, sliced after
   seeds discarded
60g/1 small banana, sliced into
   1cm-thick pieces
30g/1 passion fruit, seeds
   scooped out of shell
160g strawberries, halved
2 tsp freshly squeezed lime juice
1 tsp light brown sugar
250g plain soya or **coconut soya**
   yogurt
½ tsp vanilla extract
1 tsp poppy seeds

WHAT TO DO

1 Combine the fruit in a bowl with the lime juice and brown sugar.
2 In a separate bowl, mix the yogurt and vanilla extract together.
3 Place a spoonful of fruit into a tall glass, followed by a spoonful of yogurt and repeat (don't mix the layers). Sprinkle with the poppy seeds and serve immediately.

Preparation time: 10 minutes
Cooking time: N/A
Serves: 2

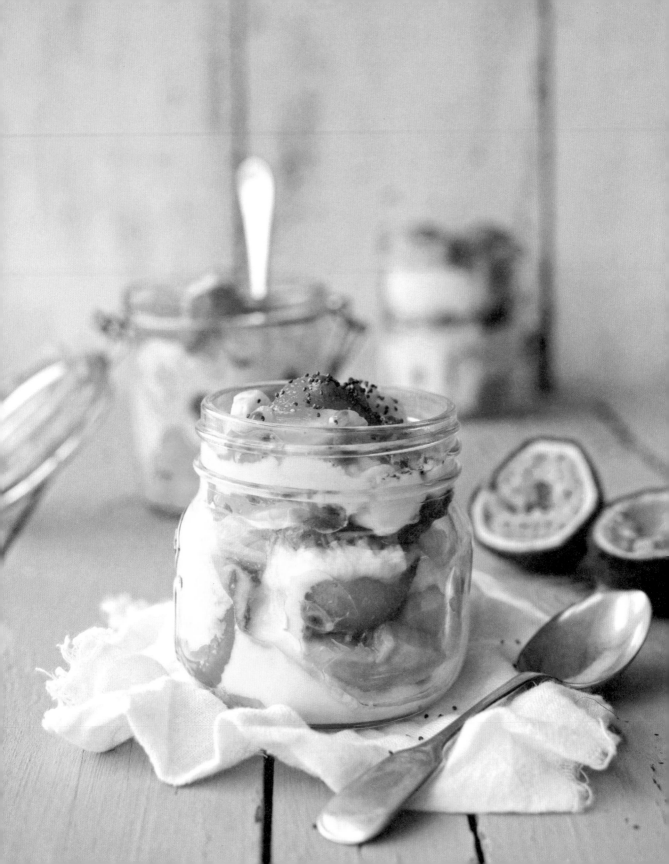

BRUNCH

Buckwheat Pancakes with Blueberry Compote

These light, crispy pancakes have a nutty flavour. Cook double the amount of compote and store the leftovers in the fridge. Stir it through some soya yogurt for another great low FODMAP breakfast or snack.

Portion size: 324g **Kcals:** 397 **Fat:** 9.8g **Saturated fat:** 3.5g **Carbs:** 58g **Sugar:** 22g **Fibre:** 6.8g **Protein:** 15.6g **Salt:** 0.4g **Allergens:** Milk, eggs

INGREDIENTS

260ml lactose-free milk

1 egg

1 tsp olive oil

pinch of salt

105g buckwheat flour

1 tbsp butter or oil, for cooking

For the blueberry compote:

1 tsp butter

1 tbsp caster sugar

½ tsp vanilla extract

200g blueberries

WHAT TO DO

1 Place the milk, egg, oil and salt into a large bowl and mix well.

2 Sift the buckwheat flour into a separate bowl. Gradually add the flour to the milk mixture, stirring constantly until a smooth batter is formed. You can also blend the batter in a blender if you prefer. Allow to rest for 30 minutes before cooking.

3 Add a small knob of butter or a drop of oil to a hot non-stick frying pan set over a medium heat. Pour in one-eighth of the batter and cook until air bubbles start to appear in the centre of the pancake. Flip the pancake and cook for another 3–4 minutes, until the bottom is nicely browned. Repeat with the remaining batter and keep the pancakes warm.

4 To make the blueberry compote, melt the butter over a low heat. Stir in the sugar and vanilla extract and cook until the sugar melts, then add the blueberries. Cook for 2–3 minutes, until the fruit starts to soften. Serve with the warm pancakes.

Preparation time: 40 minutes
Cooking time: 20 minutes
Serves: 2

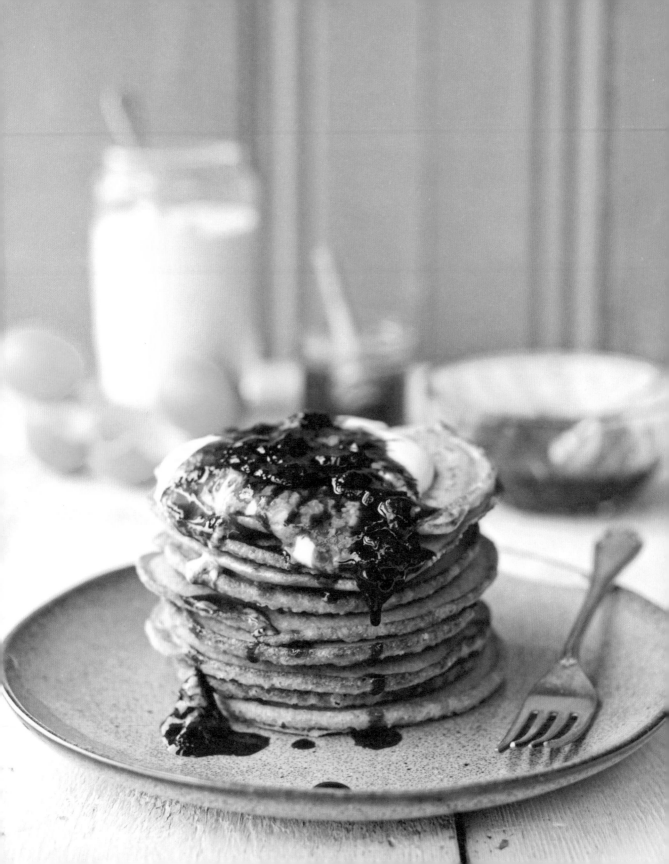

Deluxe French Toast

A fancy cheese and tomato toasted sambo!

Portion size: 299g **Kcals:** 456 **Fat:** 26g **Saturated fat:** 10.1g **Carbs:** 33g **Sugar:** 6.4g **Fibre:** 3.6g **Protein:** 19.7g **Salt:** 1.4g
Allergens: Eggs, milk, may contain sesame, may contain soya

INGREDIENTS

150g/approx. 10 cherry tomatoes

3 tsp olive oil

1 tsp fresh or dried oregano

2 eggs

120ml lactose-free milk

60g Gruyère or Cheddar, grated

1 tsp ground cinnamon

salt and freshly ground black pepper

150g/4 slices of gluten-free
    multi-seed bread

WHAT TO DO

1 Preheat the oven to 220°C.

2 Mix the tomatoes with 1 teaspoon of the oil and all of the oregano, then tip out onto a baking tray. Roast in the oven for about 15 minutes, until the skins split.

3 While the tomatoes are cooking, break the eggs into a bowl and beat lightly with a fork. Stir in the milk, cheese and cinnamon and season to taste.

4 Heat a pan coated with the remaining 2 teaspoons of oil over a medium–low heat. Place a slice of bread, one at a time, into the egg mixture, letting the bread soak for a few seconds, then carefully turn to coat the other side.

5 Transfer the bread to the pan and cook until the bottom of the bread is golden brown. Turn and brown the other side.

6 Serve the cheesy egg bread with some roasted tomatoes on top. Season with black pepper before serving.

Preparation time: 10 minutes
Cooking time: 20 minutes
Serves: 2

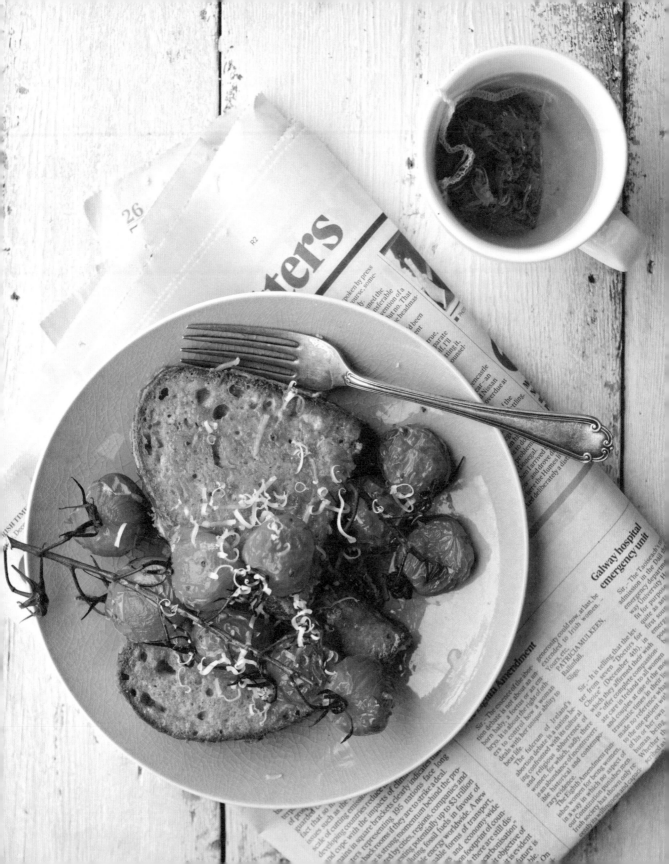

Mild Kedgeree with Raita

Kedgeree is a dish consisting of cooked flaked fish, boiled rice, parsley, hard-boiled eggs, curry powder and butter or cream. A raita is a yogurt-based condiment that usually contains vegetables. Raitas are designed to be cooling to counteract the effect of spicy dishes.

Portion size: 378g **Kcals:** 473 **Fat:** 24g **Saturated fat:** 5.8g **Carbs:** 29g **Sugar:** 3.6g **Fibre:** 2.4g **Protein:** 35g **Salt:** 1.3g **Allergens:** Fish, eggs, milk, soya

INGREDIENTS

1 tsp rapeseed oil

1 tbsp hot or mild curry powder (depending on how spicy you can tolerate)

½ tsp ground turmeric

180g/1 tin of mackerel fillets in brine, drained and patted dry with kitchen paper

160g cooked or leftover rice

2 hard-boiled eggs, cut in half

juice of ½ lemon

1 tsp butter, melted

1 tbsp chopped fresh parsley

salt and freshly ground black pepper

For the raita:

150g/⅓ cucumber, coarsely grated

125g plain soya yogurt

½ tsp ground cumin

pinch of chilli powder (optional)

WHAT TO DO

1 Heat the oil in a frying pan set over a medium heat. Add the curry powder and turmeric, then the mackerel fillets. Cook on each side for 2–3 minutes. Remove from the pan and flake into pieces, then set aside.

2 Place the cooked rice into a large bowl. Add the cooled fish along with the hard-boiled eggs, lemon juice, melted butter and fresh parsley and mix well. Season as desired.

3 To make the raita, use your hands to squeeze the excess water from the grated cucumber. Place the cucumber in a bowl and stir in the yogurt, cumin, chilli powder, if using, and some freshly ground black pepper. Cover the bowl with cling film and refrigerate until required.

4 Serve the kedgeree with the chilled raita on the side.

Preparation time: 10 minutes
Cooking time: 10 minutes
Serves: 2

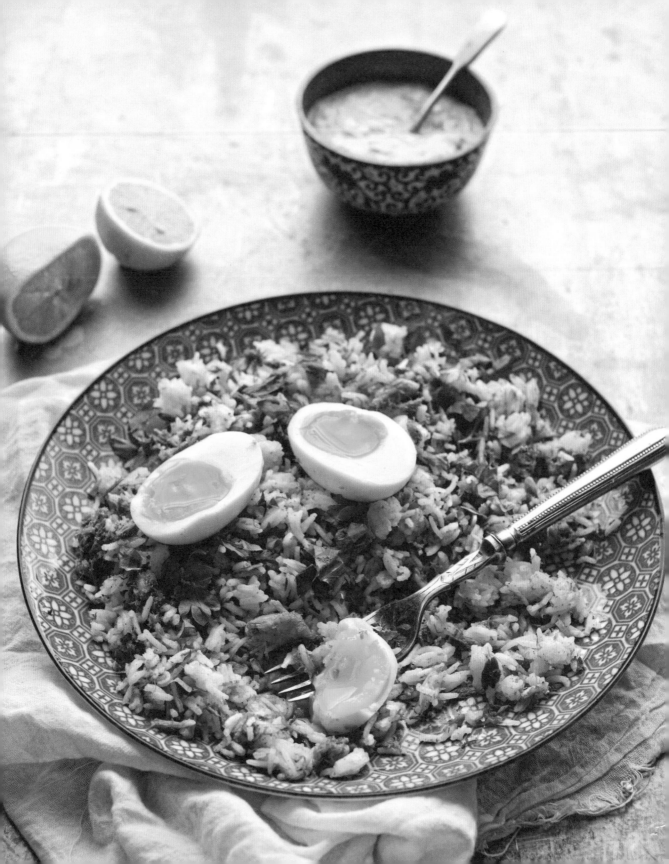

Power Omelette

This omelette has it all! A breakfast beast, but you can have it at any time of the day.

 Portion size: 378g **Kcals:** 361 **Fat:** 27g **Saturated fat:** 8.4g **Carbs:** 8.3g **Sugar:** 7.9g **Fibre:** 3.9g **Protein:** 19g **Salt:** 2.2g **Allergens:** Eggs, milk

INGREDIENTS

1½ tbsp olive oil

260g/2 medium tomatoes, diced

160g/1 red pepper, chopped into
    small pieces

1 tbsp dried herbs, such as
    Herbes de Provence

salt and freshly ground black
    pepper

4 eggs

**15g/3 spring onions (green part
    only)**, sliced

35g/approx. 2 handfuls of pitted
    black olives, halved

60g feta, crumbled

WHAT TO DO

1 Heat 1 tablespoon of the oil in an ovenproof frying pan (one
    with a lid). Add the tomatoes, pepper and dried herbs, then
    turn the heat right down to its lowest setting and season
    with salt and pepper. Put a lid on the frying pan and let it
    cook gently for about 10 minutes, until the vegetables are
    tender. Stir halfway through so they don't brown too much.

2 Break the eggs into a large bowl and whisk them lightly.
    Season well.

3 When the vegetables are cooked, add them to the eggs in
    the bowl, followed by the spring onions.

4 Put the frying pan back on a medium heat and add the
    remaining ½ tablespoon of the oil. Pour the omelette mix
    into the frying pan, then immediately turn the heat down to
    its lowest setting. Scatter the olives on top.

5 Cook the omelette for about 10–15 minutes, uncovered. Every
    now and then draw the edge in gently with a palette knife,
    as this will give it a rounded edge. Once it looks nearly set,
    sprinkle the cheese on top, then place under a hot grill and
    cook until golden and bubbling on top. The omelette should
    be cooked through but still moist in the centre.

6 Slide the omelette out of the pan, then cut into wedges.
    Serve hot or cold.

Preparation time: 15 minutes
Cooking time: 25 minutes
Serves: 2

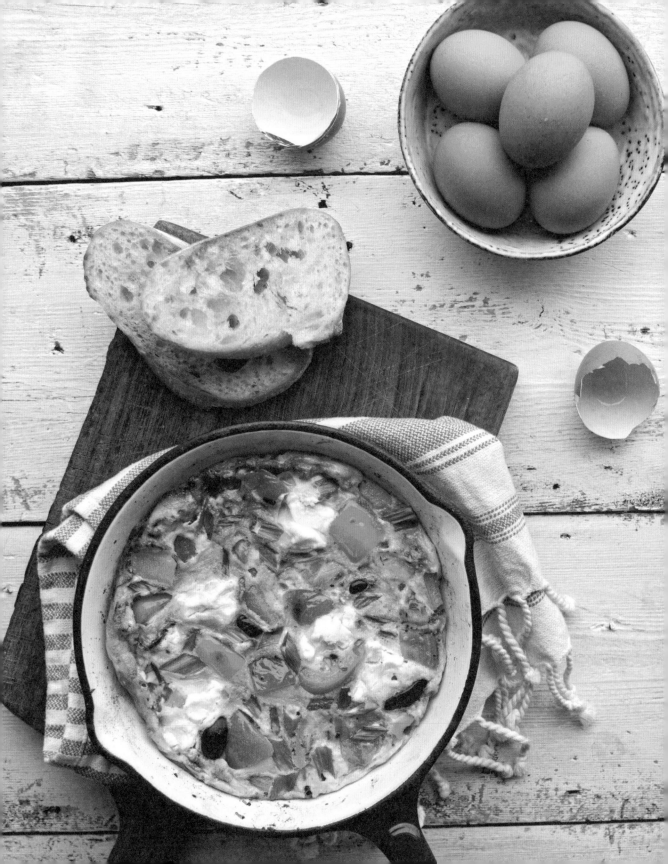

Fluffy Raspberry Pancakes

These are a massive hit with all family members! You can also use mixed berries and use extra milk if you need to thin the batter. **You may want to use Greek yogurt to serve, as 50g per serving is tolerated by most.**

  Portion size: 314g* **Kcals:** 426 **Fat:** 14.7g **Saturated fat:** 5g **Carbs:** 55g **Sugar:** 14.6g **Fibre:** 5.1g **Protein:** 15.6g **Salt:** 1.8g **Allergens:** Eggs, milk, may contain gluten, may contain soya, may contain lupin. *Analysis completed using Greek yogurt. If soya yogurt is used insead, it will contain soya instead of milk.*

INGREDIENTS

95g gluten-free flour

1 tsp baking powder

¾ tsp baking soda

pinch of salt

1 large egg, lightly beaten

230ml lactose-free milk

2 tsp butter, melted and cooled

100g fresh or frozen raspberries
(thawed if frozen), plus extra
to serve

1 tbsp olive oil

100g soya yogurt or
50g Greek yogurt

1 heaped tsp raspberry jam

WHAT TO DO

1 Whisk together the flour, baking powder and baking soda in a large bowl. Add a pinch of salt and set aside.

2 In a separate bowl, whisk together the egg, milk and melted butter. Add to the flour mixture, stirring until just combined, then fold in the raspberries.

3 Heat the oil in a pan set over a moderately high heat. Drop tablespoons of the batter onto the pan and cook for 2–3 minutes, until bubbles form on top. Turn over and cook for 1 minute on the other side.

4 Mix the yogurt and jam together and serve on top of the pancakes along with some extra raspberries.

Preparation time: 10 minutes
Cooking time: 5–10 minutes
Serves: 2

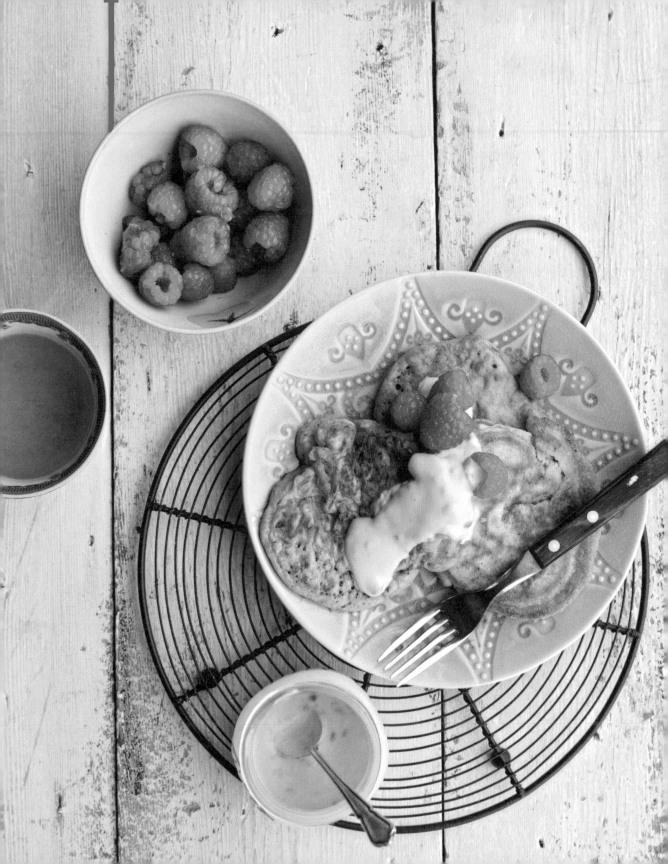

Lunch

Many people eat lunch *away* from home, so we've put together some ideas for lunches that take no more than a few *minutes* to assemble before you leave for work or college. *Batch* cooking soup or prepping veg ahead of time also makes life easier when you're *dashing* out the door.

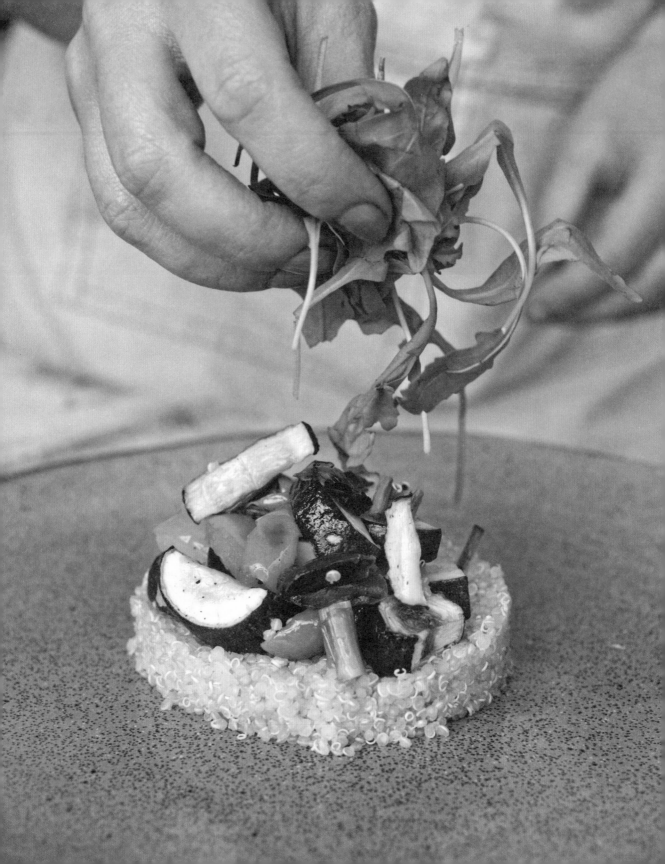

Quick lunch ideas

* Flask of fresh carrot and ginger soup (page 44) with 1 small wholemeal gluten-free roll and 1 orange

* Allowed salad topped with 1 sliced skinless chicken breast, **no more than 1 tablespoon of balsamic dressing** and 1 wholemeal gluten-free pitta

* 4 oat crackers with 2 tablespoons light soft cheese and allowed salad plus 1 pot of soya yogurt (315 calories)

* 1 small box of sushi and 1 tub of homemade fresh fruit salad (check the labels on the sushi and make sure only allowed fruit is included in the salad)

* Sandwich or wrap made with a gluten-free or corn tortilla or 100% sourdough spelt bread, filled with cooked turkey, chicken, prawns, tuna, crab, Brie, Cheddar, Swiss cheese, mozzarella, Edam, egg and lettuce, spinach, rocket, tomatoes, **<3 tablespoons sweetcorn**, cucumber, **green part of spring onion**, radish, **<4 slices of beetroot**, **<¼ avocado** with an oil and vinegar dressing, mayonnaise and/or mustard

* Chicken or prawn rice salad with cooked rice, chicken or prawns, lettuce, suitable low FODMAP salad veg and salad dressing (3:1 ratio of olive oil to balsamic vinegar – **1 tablespoon per person of balsamic vinegar is allowed**). Add 1 teaspoon mustard, lemon juice, lime juice, chopped herbs or Tabasco sauce and season with salt and pepper.

* Antipasti using low FODMAP foods: selection of cheeses, red pepper and carrot sticks, olives, grapes, strawberries, gluten-free crackers, oat cakes or breadsticks

Out to lunch

Grilled fish
with allowed salad or vegetables

Grilled skinless chicken breast
with allowed salad or vegetables

Grilled lean steak
with allowed salad or vegetables

Tuna niçoise salad
(tuna, olives, potato halves, egg, lettuce leaves and a suitable dressing)

Greek salad
(tomato, feta, olives, lettuce, suitable dressing) and a small gluten-free bread roll

Gluten-free pizza
with allowed vegetable or fruit toppings

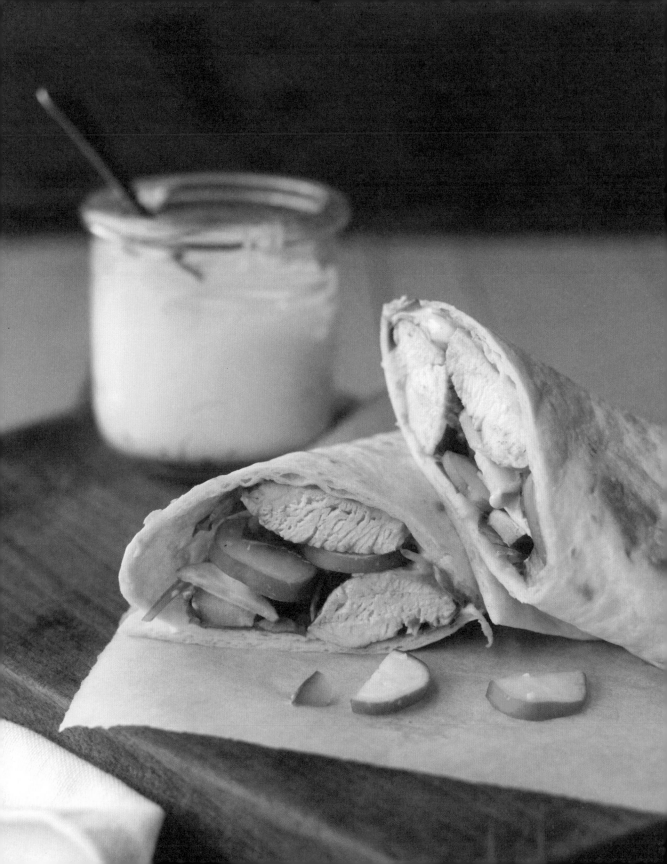

Baked Potato Ideas

The baked potato is a home favourite. There are always a few potatoes lying around and they make the perfect light meal: easy and indulgent. The best part is that there are endless toppings you can combine for new fun flavours. The recipes below are delicious, easy to make and all come in at under 400 kcals each.

BAKED POTATO WITH GRATED FARMHOUSE CHEDDAR AND MUSTARD

Portion size: 220g **Kcals:** 361 **Fat:** 16.1g **Saturated fat:** 8.9g **Carbs:** 36g **Sugar:** 4.3g **Fibre:** 4.3g **Protein:** 15.3g **Salt:** 2g **Allergens:** Gluten, mustard, milk

BAKED POTATO WITH ROAST PEPPER, BASIL AND LEMON JUICE

Portion size: 253g **Kcals:** 192 **Fat:** 0.6g **Saturated fat:** 0.2g **Carbs:** 38g **Sugar:** 6g **Fibre:** 5.9g **Protein:** 5g **Salt:** 0.02g **Allergens:** None

BAKED POTATO WITH BLUE CHEESE AND WALNUTS

Portion size: 215g **Kcals:** 400 **Fat:** 21g **Saturated fat:** 10.1g **Carbs:** 34g **Sugar:** 2.6g **Fibre:** 4.9g **Protein:** 15.1g **Salt:** 0.8g **Allergens:** Tree nuts, milk

BAKED POTATO WITH SALMON OR TUNA

Portion size: 295g **Kcals:** 385 **Fat:** 15.3g **Saturated fat:** 10.2g **Carbs:** 36.3g **Sugar:** 3.3g **Fibre:** 4.9g **Protein:** 23.1g **Salt:** 0.6g **Allergens:** Milk, fish

INGREDIENTS

210g/1 medium potato

Toppings:

grated farmhouse Cheddar (40g) and
    mustard (15g)
roast pepper (80g), 1 tsp chopped
    fresh basil leaves and
    1 tsp lemon juice
farmhouse blue cheese (40g) and
    chopped walnuts (10g)
1 tin of pink salmon or tuna mixed
    with lemon juice, black pepper and
    2 tbsp crème fraîche

WHAT TO DO

1 Place the potato in an oven preheated to 200°C and bake for 45–60 minutes or microwave for 15 minutes.
2 Pick your toppings and sprinkle them over the top.

Preparation time: 5-10 minutes
Cooking time: 15–60 minutes
Serves: 1

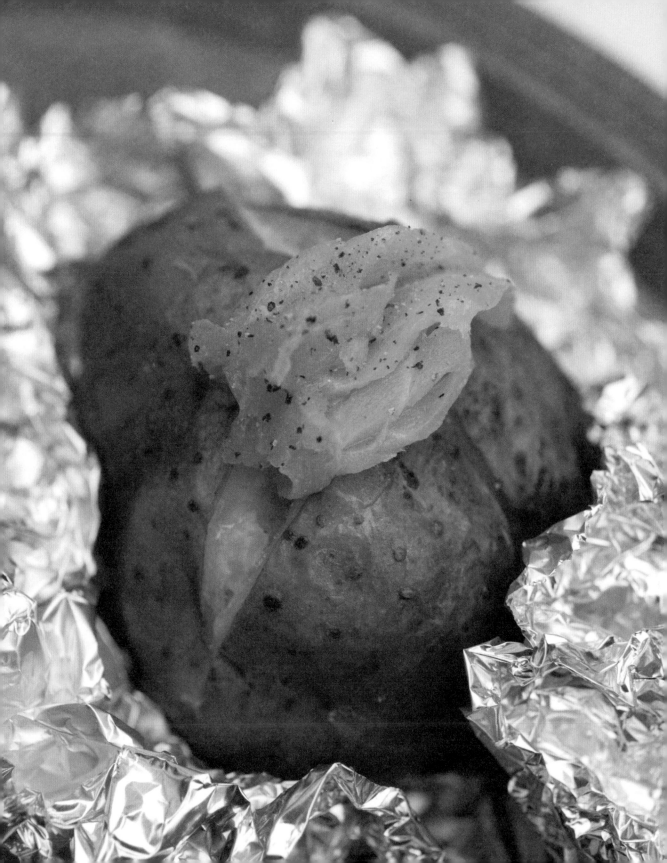

Carrot and Ginger Soup

If you're looking for a nourishing soup that's easy to make, then this is it. The sweetness of the carrot fused with the ginger and a hint of mustard makes this rich soup delightful and warm, perfect for when you're feeling a bit run down, especially in cold weather. To complete the experience, serve with 100% sourdough spelt bread. **Remember, you can eat up to 50g of natural cow's milk yogurt or Greek yogurt at a sitting as long as you don't have FODMAPs elsewhere in the meal.** Like all the soups in this chapter, this is a great option for lunch in the office.

  Serving size: 452g **Kcals:** 102 **Fat:** 1.4g **Saturated fat:** 0.5g **Carbs:** 16.3g **Sugar:** 13.8g **Fibre:** 7g **Protein:** 2.9g **Salt:** 1g **Allergens:** Celery, mustard, sesame, sulphites, may contain milk

INGREDIENTS

1 level tsp mustard powder
2.5cm piece of fresh ginger, peeled and grated
salt and freshly ground black pepper
1 litre homemade low FODMAP stock (page 118)
600g/6 medium carrots, chopped
60g/1 celery stick, finely sliced
fresh parsley, to garnish
1 tsp black or white sesame seeds, to garnish
<50g per person Greek yogurt, to serve (optional)

WHAT TO DO

1 Add the mustard powder, ginger, salt and pepper to 3 tablespoons of the stock and cook for 5 minutes, stirring. Stir in the carrots and celery, then pour in the remaining stock and simmer gently for 30–40 minutes, until the vegetables are tender. Blend until smooth.

2 Garnish with the parsley, sesame seeds and a swirl of Greek yogurt, if using.

Preparation time: 10 minutes
Cooking time: 45 minutes
Serves: 4

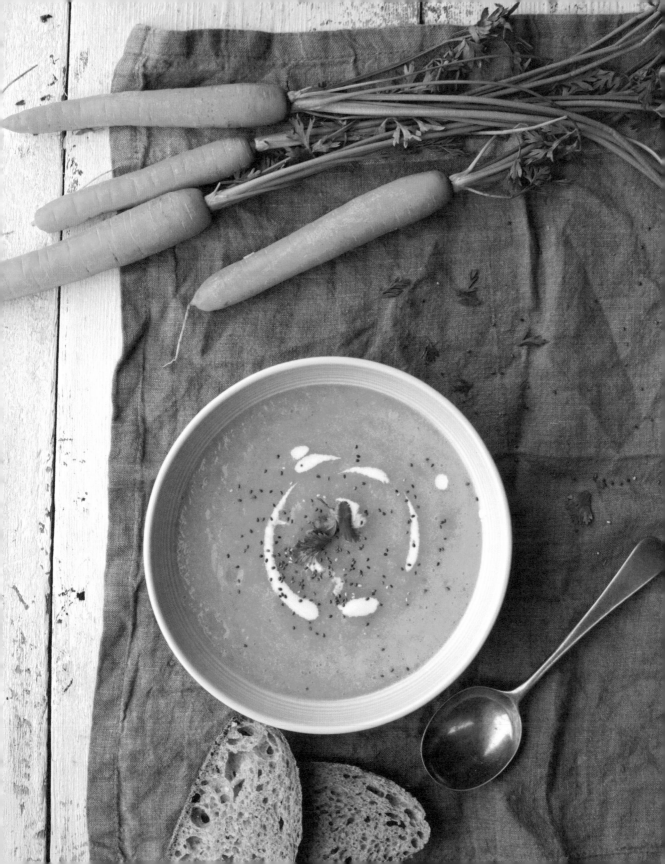

Courgette and Spinach Soup

A green favourite, this simple but delectable veggie soup is tasty and invigorating. It's also a great way to use up any extra courgettes or half-eaten bags of spinach from the salad drawer in your fridge.

Serving size: 624g **Kcals:** 229 **Fat:** 7.5g **Saturated fat:** 1.4g **Carbs:** 27g **Sugar:** 8g **Fibre:** 8.5g **Protein:** 8.2g **Salt:** 1.1g **Allergens:** Celery, milk

INGREDIENTS

2 tbsp garlic-infused olive oil

425g/2 medium potatoes, cut into 1.25cm cubes

600g courgettes, roughly chopped

1 litre homemade low FODMAP stock (page 118)

200g spinach leaves

50g/10 spring onions (green part only), chopped

juice of 1 lemon

pinch of salt

handful of fresh coriander, chopped

125g cow's milk natural yogurt

WHAT TO DO

1 Heat the olive oil in a large pot set over a medium heat, then add the chopped potatoes and courgettes. Add the stock and simmer for 10–15 minutes, until the potatoes are soft.

2 Stir in the spinach and spring onion tops and wait for them to wilt – this should only take about 10 seconds. Purée with a hand blender until smooth. Whisk in a large squeeze of lemon juice, then taste and add a pinch of salt if needed.

3 Serve with fresh coriander and a swirl of cow's milk natural yogurt.

Preparation time: 10 minutes
Cooking time: 15 minutes
Serves: 4

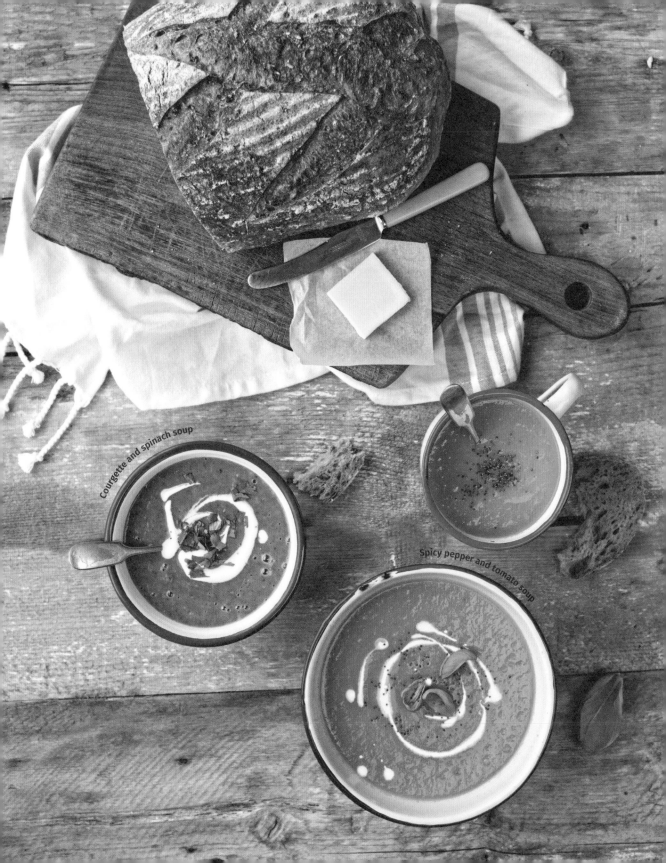

Courgette and spinach soup

Spicy pepper and tomato soup

Spicy Pepper and Tomato Soup

The blend of pepper, tomatoes and chilli makes this soup delicious and nutritious. Serve cold as a refreshing Spanish-style gazpacho or hot to warm you up on a chilly day.

Portion size: 357g **Kcals:** 70 **Fat:** 1.3g **Saturated fat:** 0.2g **Carbs:** 10.1g **Sugar:** 9.6g **Fibre:** 3.6g
Protein: 2.4g **Salt:** 0.6g **Allergens:** Celery, may contain milk

INGREDIENTS

2 tbsp garlic-infused olive oil
480g/3 red peppers, halved
2 red chillies, deseeded and chopped
2 x 400g tins of chopped tomatoes
700–900ml homemade low FODMAP
    stock (page 118)
salt and freshly ground black pepper
fresh basil leaves, to garnish
125g cow's milk natural yogurt,
    to serve (optional)

WHAT TO DO

1 Heat the olive oil in a heavy-based saucepan set over a medium heat. Add the peppers and cook gently for 15 minutes, stirring occasionally, until they are soft. Add the chopped chillies and cook for a few more seconds. Add the tomatoes, stock and seasoning and bring to the boil.

2 Take the pan off the heat and blitz the soup with a hand-held blender. Garnish with the basil and a swirl of cow's milk natural yogurt and serve straight away.

Preparation time: 10 minutes
Cooking time: 20 minutes
Serves: 6

Spicy Parsnip Soup

This is a delicious soup with aromatic flavours. You will need to use FODMAP-friendly stock (see page 119), but don't be put off by this, as it's really easy and filling, yet low in calories. **Remember to stick to the recommended portion of Greek yogurt (<50g per portion). Remember to weigh it if you aren't sure about the quantity.**

Portion size: 362g **Kcals:** 210 **Fat:** 10.3g **Saturated fat:** 3.9g **Carbs:** 20g **Sugar:** 11.9g
Fibre: 6.9g **Protein:** 5.5g **Salt:** 1.2g **Allergens:** Celery, mustard, may contain milk

WHAT TO DO

1 Heat the oil in a large pan set over a medium heat. Add the parsnips and tomatoes and cook for 5 minutes, then add the spices and cook gently for 1 minute.
2 Add the stock and bring to the boil. Lower the heat and simmer for 20–25 minutes, until the parsnips are tender. Remove from the heat and blend in a food processor or with a hand-held blender.
3 Add the chopped coriander and stir in the Greek yogurt before serving, if desired.

INGREDIENTS

2 tbsp garlic-infused olive oil
700g/4 large parsnips, peeled and cut into chunks
260g/2 large tomatoes, chopped
1 tsp ground coriander
1 tsp ground cumin
½ tsp ground turmeric
½ tsp mustard seeds
1 litre homemade low FODMAP vegetable stock (page 119)
handful of fresh coriander, chopped
<50g per person of Greek yogurt, to serve (optional)

Preparation time: 10 minutes
Cooking time: 35 minutes
Serves: 4

Smoked Mackerel Pâté

This pâté is is so easy to make and is great as a snack and at its best loaded onto toast. This recipe works well with other smoked fish too, such as trout or salmon. **A maximum serving at any one time would be 100g as the cut-off for cream cheese is 40g per serving.**

  Portion size: 58g* **Kcals:** 104 **Fat:** 7.2g **Saturated fat:** 2.4g **Carbs:** 0.8g **Sugar:** 0.6g **Fibre:** 0.1g **Protein:** 8.9g
Salt: 0.4g **Allergens:** Fish, milk, may contain eggs, may contain gluten if served with sourdough spelt bread

INGREDIENTS
225g smoked mackerel fillets
100g cream cheese
juice of ½ lemon
½ tsp cayenne pepper (optional)
½ tsp cumin powder
½ tsp freshly ground black pepper
pinch of salt
pinch of smoked paprika, to garnish
toasted 100% sourdough spelt bread,
    to serve (optional)

WHAT TO DO
1 Remove the skin from the mackerel fillets and discard any bones, then flake the flesh into a bowl. Add the cream cheese, lemon juice and spices. Mix thoroughly or gently blend until well combined, then taste and adjust the seasoning if needed.
2 Transfer to a serving bowl and garnish with a pinch of smoked paprika. Serve with spelt toast on the side.

Preparation time: 5 minutes
Cooking time: N/A
Serves: 6

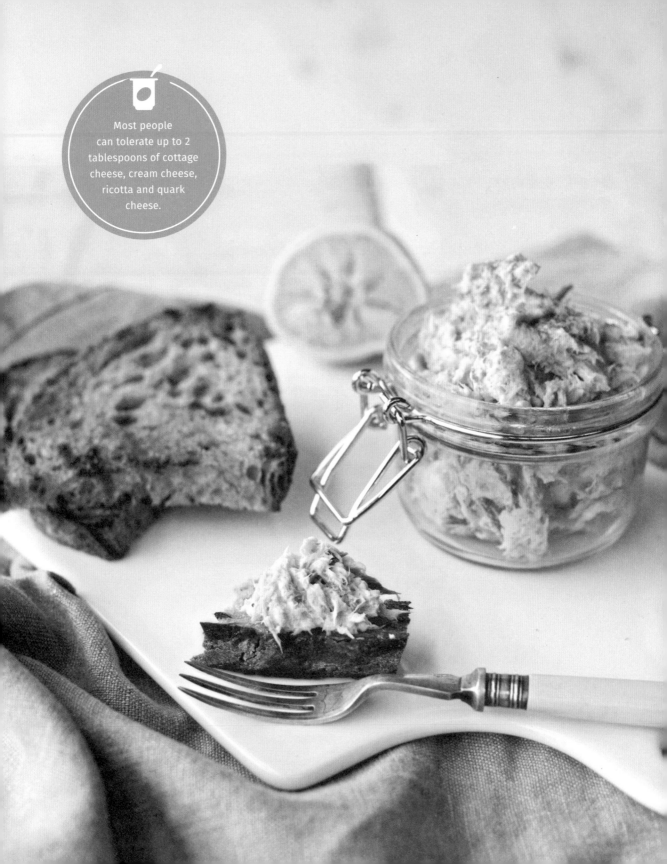

Most people can tolerate up to 2 tablespoons of cottage cheese, cream cheese, ricotta and quark cheese.

Goats' Cheese Salad with Raspberry Dressing

A great lunch or starter, this salad is sure to ignite your taste buds!

 Portion size: 224g **Kcals:** 299 **Fat:** 24g **Saturated fat:** 7.4g **Carbs:** 8.9g **Sugar:** 7.8g **Fibre:** 4.9g **Protein:** 10.3g
Salt: 0.5g **Allergens:** Tree nuts, milk, sulphites

INGREDIENTS

30g ground almonds
120g goats' cheese, cut into slices
400g mixed green salad leaves
140g cherry tomatoes, halved
60g fresh raspberries
4 tsp sunflower seeds

For the raspberry dressing:
60g fresh raspberries
1 tbsp red wine vinegar
1 tbsp maple syrup
1 tsp lemon juice
3 tbsp olive oil

WHAT TO DO

1 Preheat the oven to 180°C. Line a baking tray with non-stick baking paper.
2 Put the ground almonds on a plate, then gently roll the cheese slices in them to coat both sides. Place the coated cheese on the lined baking tray and cook in the oven for 10–15 minutes.
3 Meanwhile, toss the salad leaves, cherry tomatoes and raspberries together in a salad bowl.
4 To make the dressing, blend the raspberries with the red wine vinegar, maple syrup and lemon juice in a food processor, then slowly add the olive oil. Pour into a small jug.
5 To serve, place a large handful of salad on each plate, then top with two or three warm cheese slices. Drizzle with the raspberry dressing and sprinkle with the sunflower seeds.

Preparation time: 10 minutes
Cooking time: 15 minutes
Serves: 4

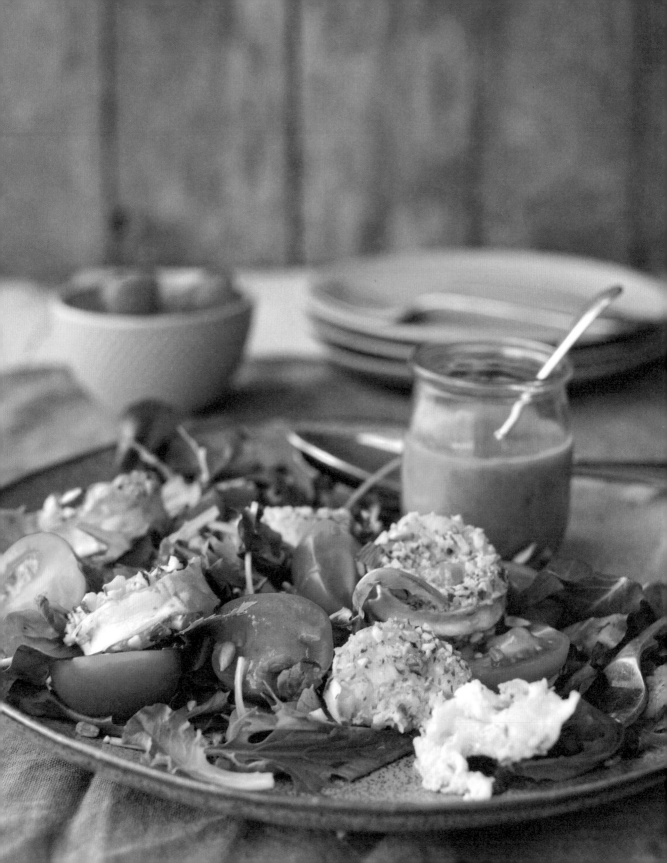

Prawn Salad with a Kick

This is a really crisp, fresh salad. You can use frozen prawns if you like, but make sure they are fully defrosted before making the salad. **Remember, only ¼ avocado is permitted per sitting.** Keep the dressing separate if you're packing this in a lunchbox.

 Portion size: 363g **Kcals:** 383 **Fat:** 27g **Saturated fat:** 4.4g **Carbs:** 8.4g **Sugar:** 7.9g **Fibre:** 3.6g **Protein:** 25g **Salt:** 2.8g **Allergens:** Crustaceans, sulphites

INGREDIENTS

150g/1 small head of butterhead
    lettuce
280g pre-cooked king prawns
160g/1 orange, cut into segments
70g/½ avocado, peeled and sliced
5g/1 spring onion (green part only),
    thinly sliced
1 tbsp chopped fresh coriander

For the chilli dressing:
1 tbsp white wine vinegar
½ tsp chilli powder (optional)
pinch of salt
3 tbsp extra virgin olive oil

WHAT TO DO

1 To make the dressing, combine the vinegar, chilli powder, if using, and the salt in a small bowl, then whisk in the oil.
2 Place some torn lettuce on one large serving platter or two individual salad plates. Arrange the prawns, orange segments and avocado over the lettuce, then sprinkle with the green part of the spring onion and the fresh coriander. Alternatively, you could serve the salad in a lettuce leaf 'cup' by using large whole leaves.
3 Drizzle the salad with the chilli dressing and serve straight away.

Preparation time: 10 minutes
Cooking time: N/A
Serves: 2

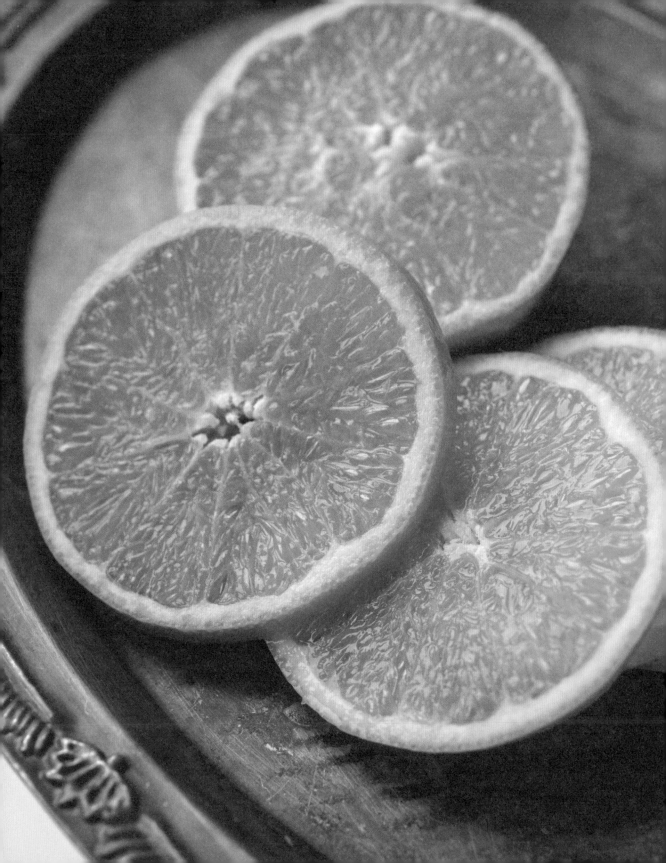

Tangy Tuna, Orange and Walnut Salad

This recipe puts a twist on your standard tuna salad. It combines citrus and walnut flavours and makes a light and scrumptious sandwich topping when you serve it with some toasted 100% sourdough spelt bread. If you don't like walnuts, add some fresh ginger and chilli flakes instead.

 Portion size: 138g **Kcals:** 165 **Fat:** 8.4g **Saturated fat:** 1.3g **Carbs:** 7.1g **Sugar:** 5.5g **Fibre:** 1.5g **Protein:** 14.7g **Salt:** 1.2g **Allergens:** Tree nuts, eggs, milk, fish

INGREDIENTS

190g tuna in sunflower oil, drained

160g/1 orange, cut into small pieces

2 heaped dessertspoons extra-light mayonnaise

50g natural cow's milk yogurt

2 dessertspoons walnuts, chopped

2 tsp ground ginger

2 tsp lemon juice

salt and freshly ground black pepper

40g/large handful of baby spinach leaves

WHAT TO DO

1 Combine the flaked tuna, chopped orange pieces, mayonnaise, yogurt, walnuts, ginger, lemon juice, salt and pepper in a bowl and mix well. Serve on a bed of baby spinach.

Preparation time: 10 minutes
Cooking time: N/A
Serves: 4

Caprese Salad

The Italian Caprese salad, aka a tomato and mozzarella salad, is the perfect dish if you want something fast. Because tomatoes taste so good with fresh basil, we've doubled up on them in this recipe! **You can use balsamic vinegar, but be sure to keep to a maximum of 1 tablespoon per portion.**

 Portion size: 407g **Kcals:** 278 **Fat:** 19.8g **Saturated fat:** 10g **Carbs:** 9.4g **Sugar:** 9.3g **Fibre:** 3.1g **Protein:** 13.5g **Salt:** 0.6g **Allergens:** Milk

WHAT TO DO

1 Mix the basil with the extra virgin olive oil in a small jug and set aside.
2 To make the salsa, mix the tomatoes, cucumber and basil together.
3 To assemble the salad, layer alternating slices of mozzarella and tomatoes around the outside of the plate. Place a large spoonful of the salsa in the middle of the plate, then pour some of the basil-infused olive oil over the salad.
4 Decorate the outside of the plate with a drizzle of balsamic vinegar, then season with salt and pepper to taste.

INGREDIENTS

approx. 5 fresh basil leaves, finely chopped
2 tsp extra virgin olive oil
1 x 120g ball of fresh mozzarella, thinly sliced
260g/2 vine-ripened tomatoes, thinly sliced
1 tbsp balsamic vinegar, for drizzling
salt and freshly ground black pepper

For the tomato salsa:
260g/2 vine-ripened tomatoes, finely diced
150g/¼ cucumber, finely diced
approx. 5 fresh basil leaves, finely chopped

Preparation time: 5 minutes
Cooking time: N/A
Serves: 2

Salad in a Jar

This is an attractive and fun way to carry your lunch to work or college. Start by getting yourself one or two glass jars with airtight lids. Make sure they are dry and clean. The idea is to layer your ingredients to build colourful concoctions of your favourite salad ingredients. There are no rules – just make sure everything is a low FODMAP food suitable for Stage 1. Anything goes, but here are some tips that might help.

BERRY GOODNESS JAR

Place 2 tablespoons of salad dressing on the bottom. Layer up mixed strawberries and blueberries, goats' cheese, sliced radishes, beansprouts, carrots, 9 almonds, flaxseeds and mixed lettuce leaves.

ITALIAN SUNSHINE JAR

Start with 2 tablespoons of salad dressing of your choice. Layer up strips of courgette, cherry tomato halves, chunks of cucumbers, small cubes of feta cheese, sliced black olives, fresh oregano, mixed lettuce leaves and toasted pine nuts.

LEMONY KALE JAR

Start with 2 tablespoons of a citrus dressing (see page 122). Layer up pineapple, blueberries, cooked chicken bites, cooked red quinoa, beansprouts and chopped kale.

SUMMER SALAD JAR

Start with 2 tablespoons of chilli lime dressing (page 123) on the bottom. Layer up halved cherry tomatoes, chopped yellow peppers, cooked brown or wild rice, small cubes of smoked halloumi (max. 50g), green parts of spring onions and fresh coriander leaves mixed with shredded Romaine lettuce.

ASIAN TOFU SALAD JAR

Start with 2 tablespoons of sesame lemon dressing (page 124). Layer up cubed firm tofu pieces, slices of red pepper, cucumber chunks, beansprouts, sunflower seeds, chopped fresh mint and baby bok choy leaves.

WHAT TO DO

1 Put your dressing at the bottom of the jar and greens at the very top. This ensures your greens stay crisp and fresh by the time you get to them.

2 With the dressing on the bottom, start by layering up vegetables such as chopped tomatoes and sliced courgettes, radishes and cucumbers.

3 Then add your protein (cheese, tofu, chicken, cold roast beef, egg).

4 Next, add drier veggies, like carrots.

5 Then add your greens, like spinach leaves or mixed lettuce leaves, and the items you want to stay crunchy on top (toasted seeds and nuts).

6 Really stuff the jar full. This helps to stop the layers from shifting and moving around, especially if the jar tips on one side in your bag.

7 Store in the fridge if possible until you're ready to eat.

8 Then all you do is shake it all about!

You can eat your salad directly out of the jar or toss it into a bowl. The dressing and toppings simply land dutifully on top of your salad leaves or greens. If you're going to savour your salad straight from the jar, you might have to eat a few mouthfuls of greens first, then shake the jar to mix it well. Don't forget to pack a fork if you're on the move.

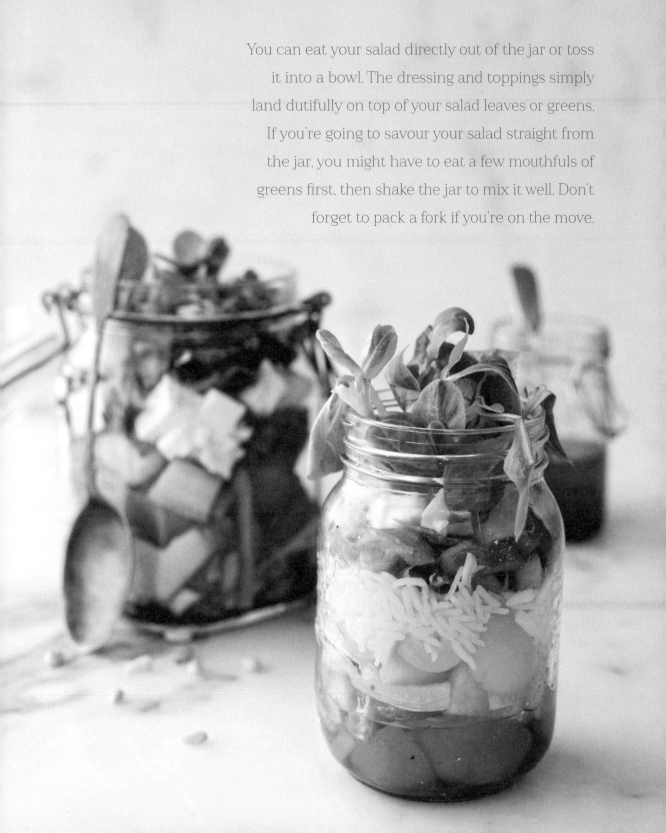

Chicken and Grape Salad with Tarragon Mayonnaise

Chicken and tarragon is the perfect match. This salad is a wonderfully quick and tasty meal or picnic idea. It's also a super way to use up last night's chicken leftovers. Allow time for this salad to sit for a while for ultimate flavour and satisfaction.

Portion size: 263g **Kcals:** 344 **Fat:** 21.3g **Saturated fat:** 6.5g **Carbs:** 5.6g **Sugar:** 5g **Fibre**: 0.7g **Protein:** 32.1g
Salt: 0.5g **Allergens:** Mustard, eggs, milk, may contain gluten

INGREDIENTS

1 x 1.5kg chicken, cooked
200g green grapes, halved and pips removed
100g extra-light mayonnaise
100ml light cream
several sprigs of fresh tarragon, leaves stripped
40g/8 spring onions (green part only), thinly sliced
salt and freshly ground black pepper
120g/1 head of lettuce or a mix of salad leaves
100% sourdough spelt bread, to serve (optional)

WHAT TO DO

1 Remove all the meat from the cooked chicken and tear into bite-size pieces. Put into a bowl with the grapes.
2 In another bowl, whisk the mayonnaise with the cream, tarragon leaves and spring onions. Pour this over the chicken and mix well, then season with salt and pepper. Allow to sit for 1 hour or so to let the flavours infuse.
3 Arrange the lettuce or salad leaves on a large serving platter and spoon over the chicken. Place in the centre of your picnic table with some crusty 100% sourdough spelt bread to serve alongside.

Preparation time: 10 minutes
Cooking time: 1 hour standing time
Serves: 8

Chicken Fried Rice

This is one of the easiest and fastest dishes to rustle up and it's probably even better than your local takeaway's fried rice! Make sure the rice is cold before stir-frying it. If you're in a hurry, you can cool rice by rinsing it in cold water.

 Portion size: 314g **Kcals:** 497 **Fat:** 14.1g **Saturated fat:** 2.6g **Carbs:** 52g **Sugar:** 1.5g **Fibre:** 3.4g **Protein:** 39g **Salt:** 1.3g **Allergens:** Gluten, eggs, sesame, soya

WHAT TO DO

1 Beat the eggs with a whisk in a bowl and season with salt and pepper. Heat 1 tablespoon of the olive oil in a large frying pan set over a medium heat. Pour the beaten eggs into the pan and leave to set for about 1 minute. It will resemble a thin omelette. Turn out onto a plate to cool, then coarsely chop into pieces. Set aside.

2 In a separate bowl, toss the chicken strips with the sesame oil and season to taste.

3 Heat the remaining tablespoon of garlic-infused olive oil in a wok or large frying pan set over a high heat. Add the chicken strips and curry powder and stir-fry for 2–3 minutes, until the chicken is lightly golden, then remove from the wok.

4 Add the green beans to the wok and stir-fry for 3–4 minutes before adding the spinach and spring onion tops. Continue to cook for another 2–3 minutes, until the spinach has wilted.

5 Stir in the cooked chicken and pre-cooked rice, sprinkle with the soya sauce and mix it all together. Remove from the heat and stir in the chopped cooked egg.

6 Divide the fried rice evenly between four bowls and garnish with additional sliced spring onion tops.

INGREDIENTS

2 large eggs, beaten

salt and freshly ground black pepper

1 tbsp garlic-infused olive oil

480g/4 boneless, skinless chicken breasts, cut into thin strips

2 tbsp sesame oil

1 tbsp curry powder

100g green beans

200g spinach

15g/3 spring onions (green part only), thinly sliced, plus extra to garnish

260g cooked basmati rice

2 tbsp low-sodium soya sauce

Preparation time: 10 minutes
Cooking time: 10 minutes
Serves: 4

Tandoori Chicken Bites

A surprisingly mildly spiced dish, perfect for a starter, lunchbox or party. It goes well with a crunchy seasonal salad. A healthy chicken nugget! **Remember to keep to the correct amount of Greek yogurt (no more than 50g per serving).**

 Portion size: 202g **Kcals:** 286 **Fat:** 14.8g **Saturated fat:** 5.9g **Carbs:** 4.5g **Sugar:** 3.7g **Fibre:** 1g **Protein:** 33g **Salt:** 0.3g **Allergens:** Milk, may contain soya

INGREDIENTS

190g full-fat Greek yogurt

2 tbsp garlic-infused rapeseed oil, plus extra for brushing

1 tbsp tomato purée

1 tsp garam masala

1 tsp paprika

1 tsp ground cumin

½ tsp chilli powder (optional)

5cm piece of fresh ginger, peeled and grated

freshly ground black pepper

480g/4 boneless, skinless chicken breasts, chopped into bite-size pieces

lime wedges, to serve

fresh coriander leaves, to garnish

WHAT TO DO

1 Mix most of the yogurt with all the ingredients except the chicken pieces in a large bowl. Add the chicken and stir until it is all well coated in the marinade. Cover the bowl with cling film and refrigerate for at least 2 hours or overnight.

2 Preheat the grill to a medium–high heat. Soak 8 wooden skewers in cold water for 15 minutes.

3 Thread the chicken onto the skewers, then place under the grill and cook, turning and brushing with oil at least once, for 10–15 minutes, until the chicken is cooked through.

4 Serve hot with lime wedges and fresh coriander leaves and the rest of the yoghurt as a dip on the side.

Preparation time: 2 hours (to marinate)
Cooking time: 15 minutes
Serves: 4

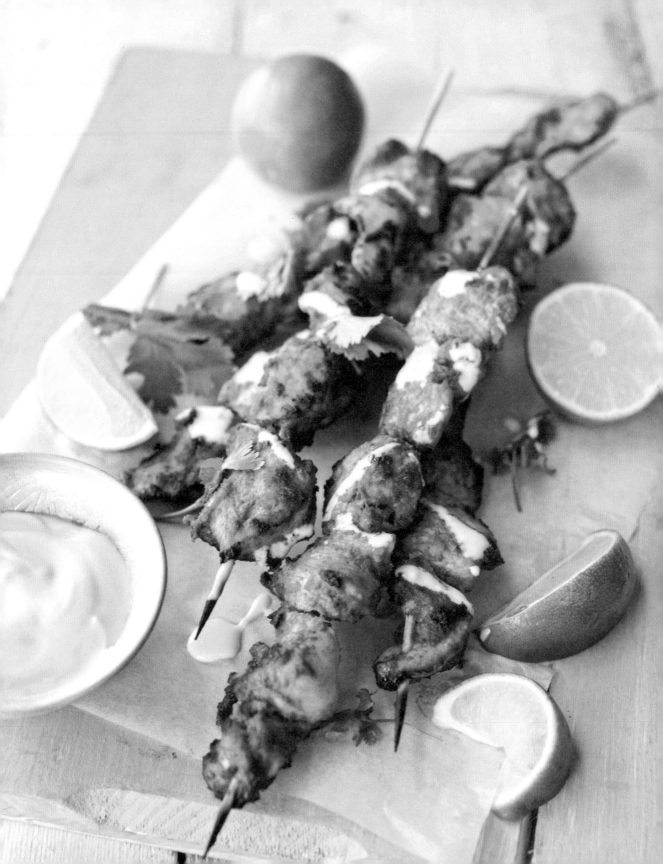

Chilli and Coriander Fish Bites

These delicious fish bites will get your taste buds jumping. They are delicious served with this homemade chilli and coriander sauce and some baby spinach leaves or a watercress salad. You can also serve them with rice or buckwheat noodles. Watch out, though, as some brands of Japanese soba noodles contain wheat. Make sure you buy 100% buckwheat noodles or rice noodles.

  Portion size: 291g **Kcals:** 215 **Fat:** 5.5g **Saturated fat:** 1g **Carbs:** 9.4g **Sugar:** 6.3g **Fibre:** 1.7g **Protein:** 31g **Salt:** 3g **Allergens:** Eggs, fish, may contain sulphites

INGREDIENTS

600g whiting, skinned, boned and
    diced
120g green beans, trimmed and
    chopped
handful of fresh basil leaves
2 tbsp fish sauce
2 tbsp red curry paste (page 134)
grated rind of 1 lemon
freshly ground black pepper
1 egg, lightly beaten
1 tbsp olive oil

For the chilli and coriander sauce:
120ml rice wine vinegar
20g light brown sugar
1 red chilli, deseeded and finely
    chopped
pinch of salt
handful of fresh coriander
60ml water
1 tsp cornflour
55g/4–5cm piece of cucumber,
    chopped

WHAT TO DO

1 Put the whiting, green beans and basil in a food processor and whizz until just combined – you don't want it to be too smooth. Transfer to a bowl and add the fish sauce, red curry paste, lemon rind and black pepper. Mix well, then add the beaten egg. Shape into eight fish cakes about 2cm thick.

2 Heat the oil in a large frying pan set over a medium heat and add half of the fish cakes. Fry gently for about 10 minutes, turning them over halfway through, until they are golden on both sides and cooked through. Cover with foil and keep warm while you cook the remaining fish cakes.

3 Make the sauce by putting the rice wine vinegar, light brown sugar, chilli and salt in a saucepan. Chop up the coriander stalks and add them to the saucepan, but keep the leaves to use later. Heat gently until the sugar dissolves.

4 Combine the water and cornflour in a separate small bowl, then stir this into the sauce. Gently simmer until the sauce thickens. Set aside to cool, then add the cucumber and chopped coriander leaves.

5 Serve the warm fish cakes with a small bowl of sauce on the side.

Preparation time: 15 minutes
Cooking time: 20 minutes
Serves: 4

Cumin and Coriander Potato Patties

Make these and pretend you are standing in the streets of Mumbai munching on a street snack!
Remember, though, that peas are a moderately high FODMAP food and only 18g are permitted per sitting. These are best served with a green salad.

Portion size: 111g **Kcals:** 154 **Fat:** 6.5g **Saturated fat:** 0.6g **Carbs:** 18.7g **Sugar:** 2.7g **Fibre:** 3.3g
Protein: 3.1g **Salt:** 0.1g **Allergens:** May contain eggs, may contain milk, may contain soya, may contain lupin

WHAT TO DO

1 Preheat the oven to 75°C.
2 Bring a pan of water to the boil. Add the potatoes and boil for 15 minutes, until tender. Drain well and set aside.
3 Meanwhile, bring another pan of water to the boil. Add the peas and boil for 2–3 minutes, until tender. Drain well, mash and set aside.
4 Soak the bread in a bowl of cold water for 5 minutes while the vegetables are boiling, then squeeze out as much of the water from the bread as possible. Place it in a bowl with the potatoes, peas, grated courgette, spring onions, spices, ginger and fresh coriander. Mix and mash together with a wooden spoon.
5 Wet your hands slightly and roll the potato mixture into balls of equal size, then flatten them until they are about 1cm thick. This makes about eight patties.
6 Heat the oil in a frying pan set over a medium heat. Fry each patty for about 4 minutes, turning once, until golden brown and crisp on both sides. Remove from the pan, drain well on kitchen paper and keep warm in the oven until you're ready to serve.

INGREDIENTS

100g floury potatoes, peeled and chopped
72g frozen peas, thawed
62g/2 slices of gluten-free bread
60g/½ courgette, grated
10g/2 spring onions (green part only), finely chopped
½ tsp ground cumin
½ tsp ground coriander
¼ tsp chilli powder, if tolerated
2cm piece of fresh ginger, peeled and grated
handful of coriander leaves, finely chopped
4 tsp rapeseed oil

Preparation time: 10 minutes
Cooking time: 30 minutes
Serves: 4

Spinach, Red Pepper and Tomato Strata

Strata, which means 'layers', is a bread, egg and veggie casserole. It can be made the night before and left in the fridge overnight so that the flavours infuse. We prefer this dish straight from the oven, but you can pop the leftovers in a lunchbox too. Sprinkle Parmesan shavings and sliced olives over the top for additional flavour.

 Portion size: 326g **Kcals:** 368 **Fat:** 10.9g **Saturated fat:** 2.5g **Carbs:** 47g **Sugar:** 6.5g **Fibre:** 4.3g **Protein:** 19.2g
Salt: 1.5g **Allergens:** Gluten, eggs, milk, may contain soya

INGREDIENTS

4 eggs
150g cow's milk natural yogurt
150ml water
1 tbsp rapeseed oil
1 heaped tsp Herbes de Provence
   or a fresh herb of your choice
salt and freshly ground black
   pepper
140g/12 cherry tomatoes, halved
160g/1 red pepper, diced
120g/1 bag of baby spinach
   leaves
300g 100% sourdough spelt
   bread, torn into pieces

WHAT TO DO

1 Preheat the oven to 180°C. Grease a 20cm x 15cm baking dish.
2 Mix the eggs, yogurt, water and oil in a bowl, then stir in the herbs and some salt and pepper.
3 In a separate bowl, mix together the tomatoes, red pepper and baby spinach leaves. Remove the stalks from the spinach leaves if they are long, chop them and add to the bowl.
4 Layer the bottom of the greased baking dish with half of the bread pieces. Place the spinach, peppers and tomatoes over this layer of bread, then cover with a top layer of bread.
5 Pour the liquid ingredients evenly over the bread, then bake in the oven for 30 minutes. Place under the grill for 2–3 minutes to crisp the top, then allow to cool so the centre sets. Serve warm or cold.

Preparation time: 10 minutes
Cooking time: 40 minutes
Serves: 4

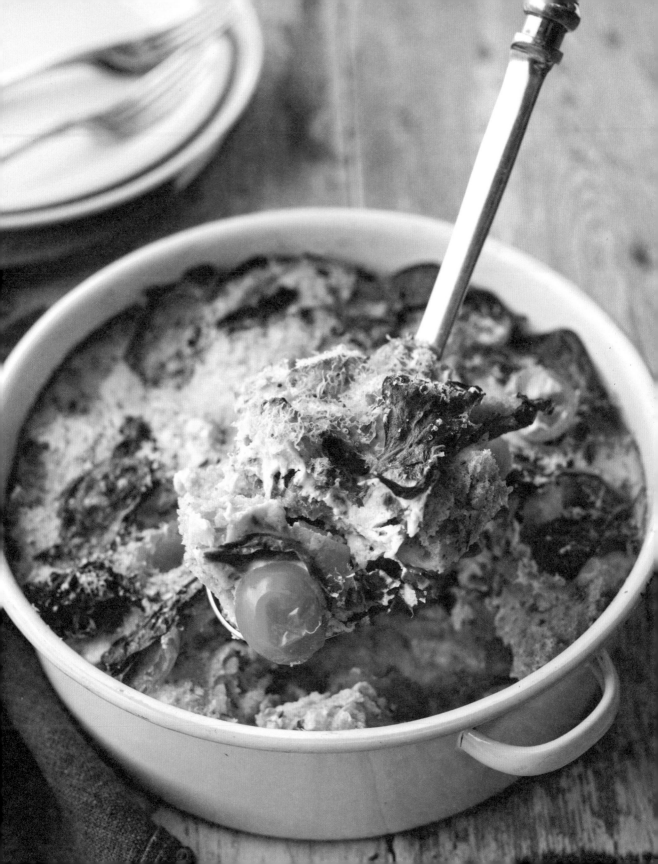

Quinoa Stack with Roasted Vegetables

Quinoa is a perfect wheat-free alternative to starchy grains. It has become popular recently, but it has actually been grown and used in South America for thousands of years. It is often used in place of starchy grains but it belongs to the same family as beets and spinach. Served with roasted vegetables in stacks, this is an elegant and tasty dish.

Portion size: 341g **Kcals:** 286 **Fat:** 14.2g **Saturated fat:** 2.6g **Carbs:** 26.3g **Sugar:** 8.6g **Fibre:** 7.4g
Protein: 9.2g **Salt:** 1.2g **Allergens:** Celery, milk, may contain sulphites

INGREDIENTS

150g quinoa
400ml homemade low FODMAP stock (page 118)
1 tbsp olive oil
salt and freshly ground black pepper
300g courgette, sliced into 1cm rings
160g/1 red pepper, chopped
160g/1 yellow pepper, chopped
40g black olives, chopped
50g/10 spring onions (green part only), chopped
2 tbsp garlic-infused olive oil
15g rocket
15g Parmesan shavings

For the dressing:
2 tbsp extra virgin olive oil
1 tbsp balsamic vinegar

WHAT TO DO

1 Preheat the oven to 170°C.
2 Place the quinoa in a fine-mesh sieve and rinse it under cold running water, rubbing your fingers through it until the water through the sieve runs clear. Place the washed quinoa in a saucepan and cover with the stock. Bring to the boil, then reduce the heat and simmer for 10 minutes, until the liquid has all been absorbed, stirring occasionally to prevent it from sticking. Drizzle with a tablespoon of olive oil and lightly season. Set aside and keep warm.
3 Mix the courgette, peppers, olives and spring onions with the garlic-infused olive oil and season with salt and pepper. Place on a baking tray and roast in the oven for 30 minutes, stirring once or twice to stop it from burning. The vegetables are ready when the pepper is soft to touch.
4 Combine the dressing ingredients with a pinch of salt and pepper. Just before serving, toss the rocket lightly through the dressing.
5 To serve, place a metal ring in the centre of each plate and half-fill with quinoa, pressing it lightly into the ring. Finish filling the ring with roasted vegetables, then carefully remove the ring. Rest some dressed rocket leaves over the top and sprinkle with Parmesan shavings.

Preparation time: 15 minutes
Cooking time: 30–40 minutes
Serves: 4

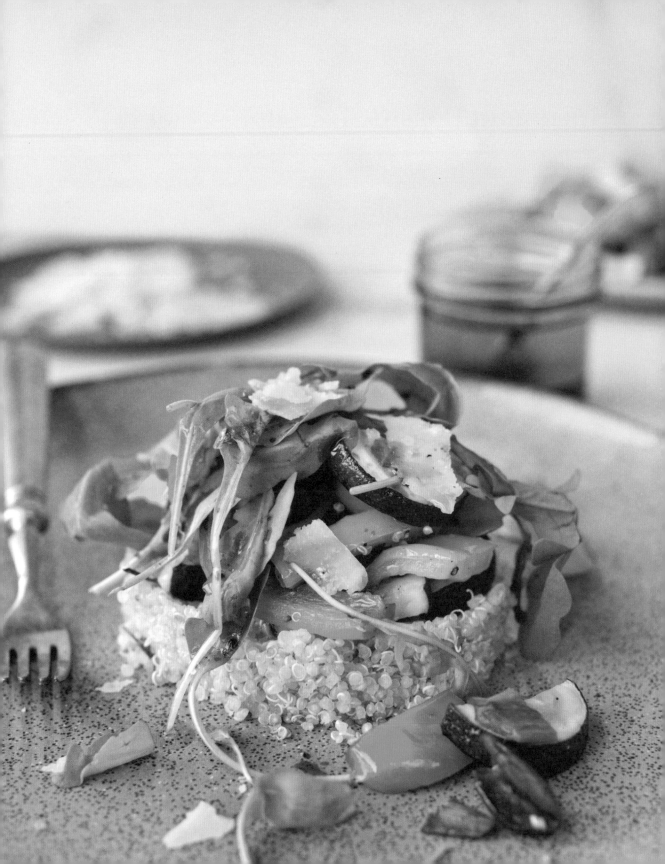

Piedmont Roasted Peppers

This recipe has an exciting Mediterranean flavour and it's very nutritious too. What's not to love? It's so easy to assemble and is the perfect dish for a light lunch, starter or lunchbox summer salad.

 Portion size: 355g **Kcals:** 392 **Fat:** 33g **Saturated fat:** 8.5g **Carbs:** 11.6g **Sugar:** 10.9g **Fibre:** 5.1g **Protein:** 9.5g
Salt: 0.5g **Allergens:** Milk, fish

INGREDIENTS

640g/4 red peppers
520g/4 plum tomatoes, skinned
    and halved lengthways
24g/8 tinned anchovy fillets, drained
    (or capers, black olives or basil)
8 tbsp garlic-infused olive oil
freshly ground black pepper
1 x 125g ball of buffalo mozzarella,
    sliced (optional)
chopped fresh parsley or fresh basil
    leaves, to garnish

WHAT TO DO

1 Preheat the oven to 180°C.
2 Cut the peppers in half lengthways and trim the pith, but try to leave the stalks on as it looks more appetising. Place the peppers in a roasting tin, cut side up, and place a skinned and halved tomato in each one. Place an anchovy fillet over each tomato, drizzle with the oil and season with pepper.
3 Bake in the oven for up to 40 minutes, until the peppers are tender. If using the mozzarella, top each halved pepper with a small slice and place back in the oven until it has melted.
4 Serve hot or cold with the juices from the roasting tin poured over. Garnish with parsley or fresh basil leaves.

Preparation time: 10 minutes
Cooking time: 40 minutes
Serves: 4

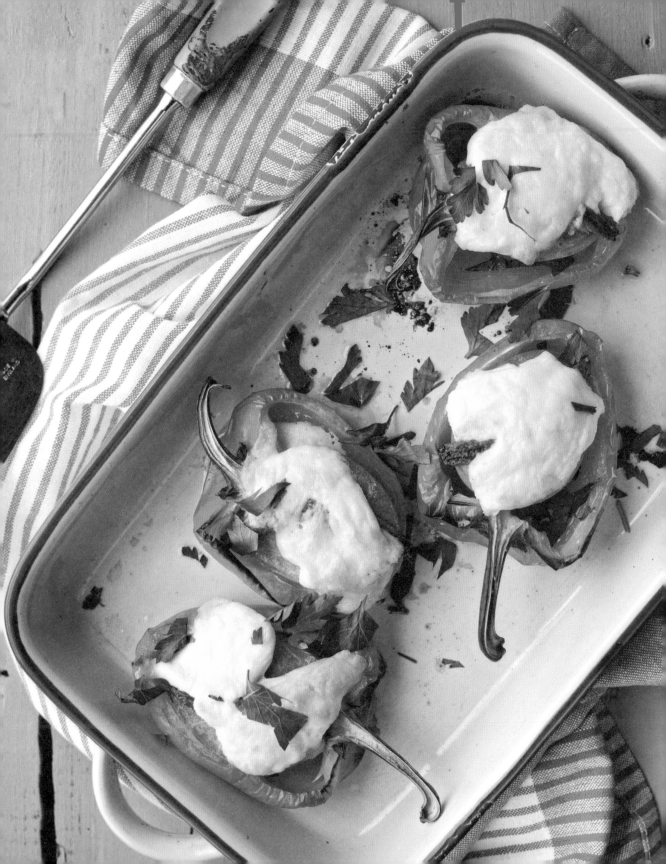

Cheesy Courgette Boats

These cheesy courgette boats are light in terms of calories, yet full of flavour. This is also a great way of using up the ends of that loaf of 100% sourdough spelt bread that you haven't got around to using. Instead of throwing it out, whizz it into breadcrumbs and freeze them if you're not using them straight away.

Portion size: 262g **Kcals:** 359 **Fat:** 19.9g **Saturated fat:** 4.9g **Carbs:** 25g **Sugar:** 4.9g **Fibre:** 5.7g **Protein:** 17.1g
Salt: 1.2g **Allergens:** Tree nuts, eggs, milk, may contain soya

INGREDIENTS

700g/8 small or 4 large courgettes

2 tsp olive oil, plus extra to grease

1 egg, beaten

½ tsp dried mixed herbs

40g ground almonds

110g grated Cheddar or Gruyère

salt and freshly ground black pepper

110g gluten-free breadcrumbs

chopped fresh parsley, to garnish

WHAT TO DO

1 Preheat the oven to 180°C. Lightly grease a baking tray.

2 Halve the courgettes lengthways. Scoop out the seeds and most of the flesh and put to one side, making sure you leave enough skin and flesh on the courgette boat to hold its shape once cooked. Chop the reserved flesh, squeezing it in your hands to extract the excess water, and set aside.

3 Place the courgette boats on the greased baking tray, hollow side down, and roast in oven for 10 minutes to soften them. Remove from the oven and allow to cool.

4 Heat the olive oil in a frying pan set over a medium heat. Add the chopped courgette flesh and cook for 5 minutes.

5 Combine the cooked courgette in a bowl with the beaten egg and herbs, then stir in the ground almonds, half of the cheese and some salt and pepper. Turn the boats right side up and spoon in the filling.

6 Combine the remaining cheese and breadcrumbs to use as a topping, sprinkling it over each courgette boat. Return to the oven for a further 20 minutes, until golden brown. Garnish with chopped fresh parsley and serve.

Preparation time: 10 minutes
Cooking time: 40 minutes
Serves: 4

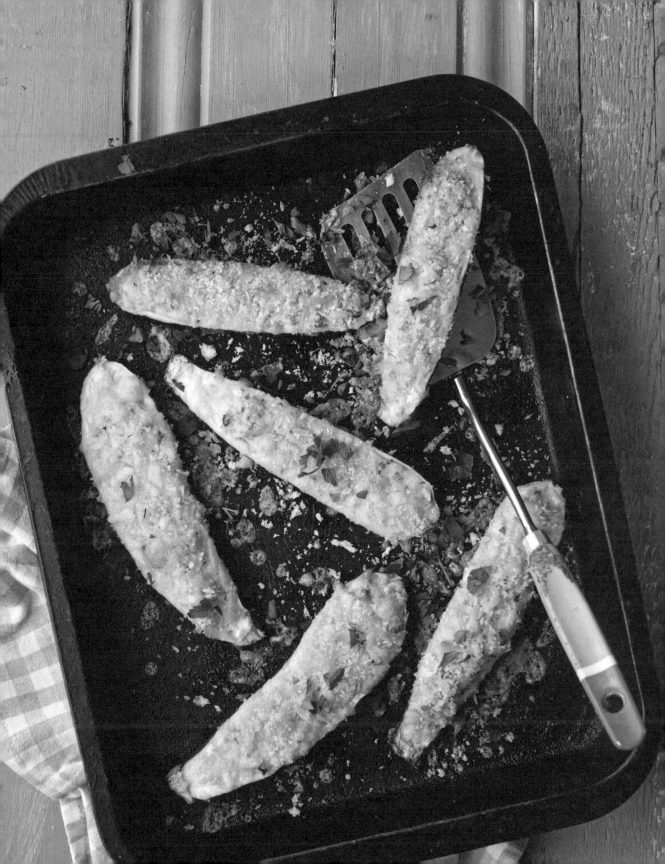

Mexican Eggs in a Pan

Simple, easy to make and packed full of flavour, this dish can be whipped up in a flash. Sprinkle with freshly chopped coriander leaves and chilli flakes for additional flavour and heat. Perfect as a light lunch or a relaxing weekend brunch.

  Portion size: 261g **Kcals:** 133 **Fat:** 7.5g **Saturated fat:** 1.8g **Carbs:** 6.1g **Sugar:** 6g **Fibre:** 2.5g **Protein:** 8.7g **Salt:** 0.2g **Allergens:** Eggs

INGREDIENTS

1 tbsp garlic-infused olive oil
68g/8 ripe tomatoes, chopped
50g/10 spring onions (green part only), chopped
1 chilli, deseeded and chopped
½ tsp ground cumin
salt and freshly ground black pepper
4 eggs
1 tbsp chopped fresh coriander

WHAT TO DO

1 Heat the olive oil in a frying pan set over a medium heat. Add the tomatoes, spring onions and chilli and cook gently for 5–6 minutes. Add the cumin and season with a pinch of salt and as much pepper as you like.
2 Break an egg over the vegetables in each quarter of the pan and cook to your liking. When the eggs are done, sprinkle with the chopped coriander and serve straight away.

Preparation time: 10 minutes
Cooking time: 15 minutes
Serves: 4

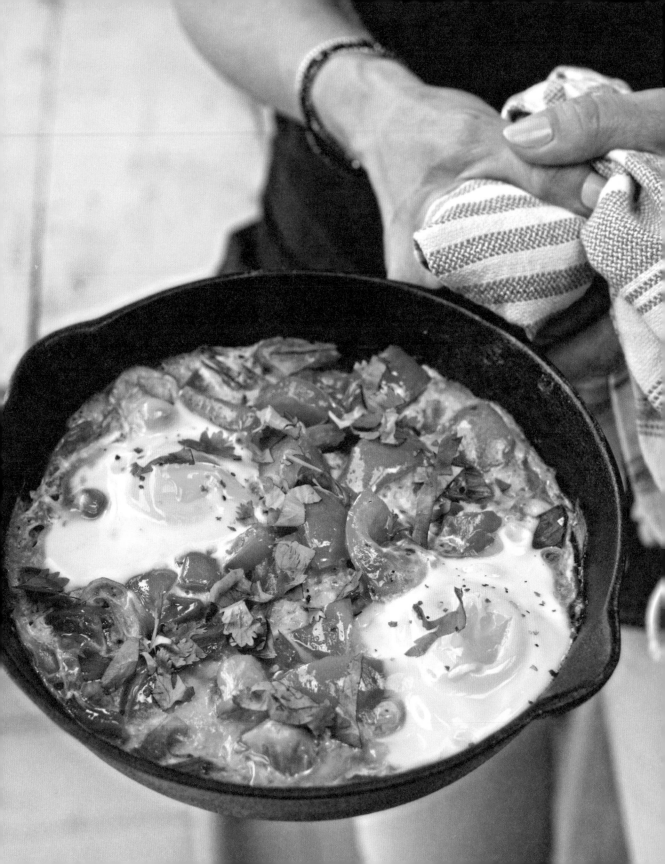

Crustless Quiche

A clever take on the original quiche Lorraine, great for a self-service family meal.

 Portion size: 280g **Kcals:** 276 **Fat:** 14.7g **Saturated fat:** 5.6g **Carbs:** 17.7g **Sugar:** 4.8g **Fibre:** 1.9g **Protein:** 17.2g
Salt: 1.1g **Allergens:** Eggs, milk, may contain gluten, may contain soya, may contain lupin

INGREDIENTS

1 tbsp garlic-infused oil
250g spinach
4 eggs
60g gluten-free flour
1 tbsp fresh thyme
½ tsp baking powder
salt and freshly ground black pepper
300ml lactose-free milk
200g cherry tomatoes, halved
30g grated Cheddar
30g grated Parmesan
handful of rocket, to garnish

WHAT TO DO

1 Preheat the oven to 180°C. Grease a flan tin or quiche dish.
2 Heat the oil in a frying pan set over a medium heat and add the spinach. Sauté until the spinach has wilted, stirring all the time. Remove from the heat and allow to cool.
3 In a large bowl, mix together the eggs, flour, thyme and baking powder. Season, then whisk in the milk.
4 When the spinach is cool, chop it into small pieces and stir it into the egg mixture. Pour the filling into the prepared tin or dish, but don't overfill! Top with most of the tomatoes, keeping some back as garnish, and both cheeses.
5 Bake in the oven for 30–35 minutes, until the quiche is set and golden. Garnish with the remaining cherry tomatoes and the rocket.

Preparation time: 15 minutes
Cooking time: 40 minutes
Serves: 4

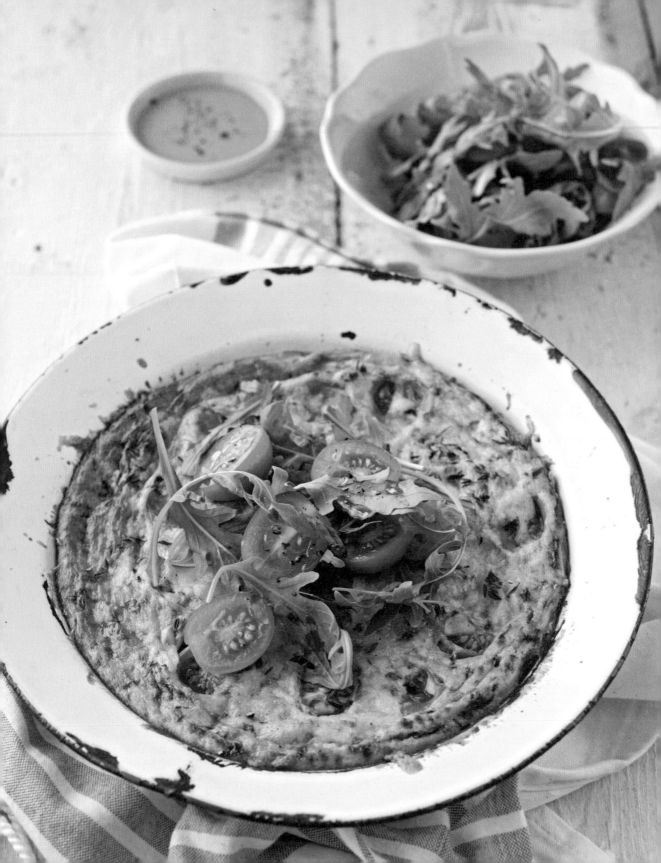

Veg Risotto with Mediterranean Salad

Making a good risotto is easy – as long as you don't forget to keep stirring! **Remember that only ½ celery stick is recommend per sitting.**

 Portion size: 477g **Kcals:** 469 **Fat:** 15.5g **Saturated fat:** 5.8g **Carbs:** 60g **Sugar:** 7.4g **Fibre:** 4g **Protein:** 12.7g **Salt:** 1.5g
Allergens: Celery, milk, sulphites

INGREDIENTS

1 litre homemade low FODMAP stock
    (page 118)
2 tbsp garlic-infused oil
15g/1 tbsp butter
pinch of asafoetida powder
120g/1 large carrot, finely diced
60g/1 stick of celery, finely diced
400g Arborio rice
250ml/2 small glasses of dry
    white wine
100g grated Parmesan
freshly ground black pepper

For the salad:
390g/3 plum tomatoes, diced
300g/½ cucumber, diced
150g mixed lettuce leaves or rocket
15 olives, quartered
15 fresh basil leaves, torn into pieces
1½ tbsp olive oil

WHAT TO DO

1 Heat the stock in a saucepan and keep it on a low heat while you're cooking the risotto.
2 Heat the garlic-infused oil and butter in a separate saucepan set over a low heat. Add the asafoetida powder, followed by the carrot and celery. Cook slowly for about 15 minutes, until soft. Add the rice and increase the heat to medium. Stir for 1–2 minutes, then add the wine and stir until it has been absorbed into the rice.
3 Begin adding the stock one ladle at a time, stirring frequently. Wait until it has all been absorbed into the rice before adding the next ladleful of stock. It takes 15–20 minutes to cook the rice. The ideal risotto is soft but still has a bite. Use extra boiling water if you run out of stock. Remove from the heat when it's done and stir in the grated Parmesan and black pepper.
4 Prepare the salad by combining all the ingredients in a large bowl and serve with the risotto.

Preparation time: 15 minutes
Cooking time: 35 minutes
Serves: 6

Zesty Quinoa Salad with Hard-Boiled Eggs

Quinoa is a healthy, quick-cooking alternative to grain. This is a fresh take on tabbouleh. It's a great accompaniment to cooked meat but it's also a good lunchbox filler.

 Portion size: 523g **Kcals:** 460 **Fat:** 17.1g **Saturated fat:** 2.9g **Carbs:** 50g **Sugar:** 8.9g **Fibre:** 8.2g **Protein:** 22g **Salt:** 0.9g **Allergens:** Eggs

WHAT TO DO

1 First rinse the quinoa in cold running water to remove its bitter coating. Heat the oil in a saucepan set over a medium heat, then add the quinoa to toast it for 6–8 minutes before adding the water. Bring to the boil, then reduce the heat and simmer for about 15 minutes or cook as per the packet instructions. Fluff up with a fork when the quinoa is cooked, then transfer to a serving bowl and allow to cool.
2 Combine all the other ingredients with the cooked quinoa. Season to taste with more pepper, oil or lemon if desired. Serve cold.

INGREDIENTS

180g uncooked quinoa, rinsed
1 tbsp garlic-infused olive oil
400ml water
225g/1/3 cucumber, finely diced
80g/1/2 red pepper, finely diced
15g/3 spring onions (green part only), finely sliced
2 hard-boiled eggs, coarsely chopped
handful of fresh mint, finely chopped
handful of fresh coriander, finely chopped
1 tbsp lemon juice
salt and freshly ground black pepper

Preparation time: 15 minutes
Cooking time: 25 minutes
Serves: 2

Dinner

You won't always want to spend *time* preparing healthy meals, especially when you get home from work or college, so many of the dinner *ideas* in this chapter are ready in less than 20 minutes. But for days when you have *more time*, there are recipe options for dinners that are a bit more *labour* intensive. There are also meals that you might never have guessed were part of a *special* diet!

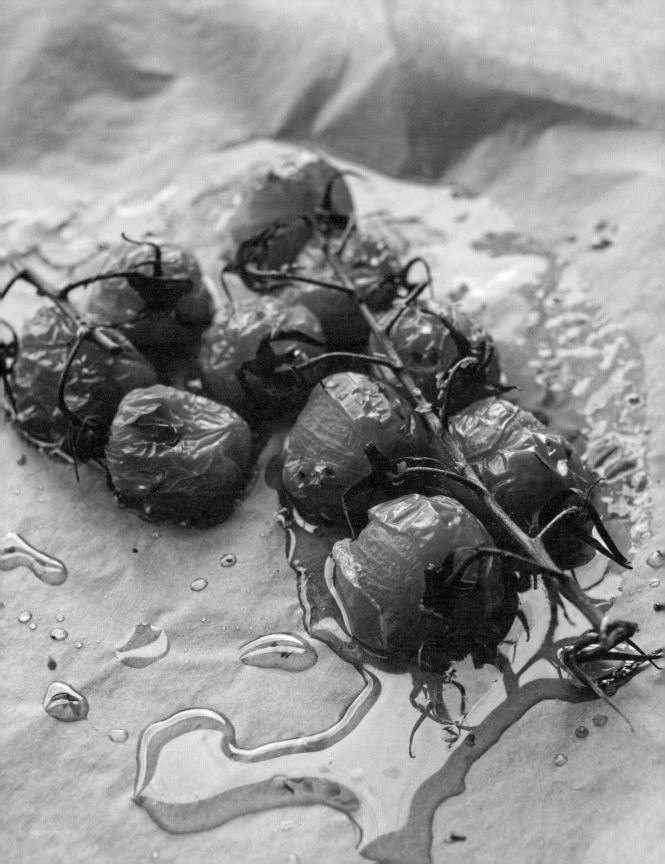

Quick dinner ideas

Providing flavoursome meals without a garlic clove or an onion in sight shouldn't put you off cooking for family and friends. Instead, invest in some garlic-, chilli- and lemon-infused oils and don't forget a pinch of asafoetida powder too.

* 1 grilled lean lamb loin chop with minted new potatoes, mixed allowed vegetables and mint sauce
* Chicken quinoa made from quinoa cooked according to the packet instructions, green part of spring onions, lemon juice, black pepper, coriander and skinless chicken breast, served with allowed salad

When you have a little more time on a Sunday, you can try ...

* Irish stew with beef, carrots, parsnips, potato, parsley and low FODMAP stock
* Meat, potatoes and veg: roast chicken, roast potatoes with suitable low FODMAP veg and gravy
* Gluten-free pizza base with low FODMAP vegetable toppings, olives and cheese

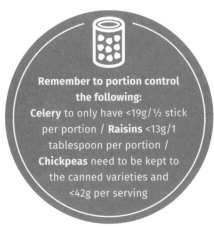

Remember to portion control the following:
Celery to only have <19g/ ½ stick per portion / **Raisins** <13g/1 tablespoon per portion / **Chickpeas** need to be kept to the canned varieties and <42g per serving

Moroccan-Inspired Lamb Tagine

A spicy, fruity and exotic dish. It takes time to cook, but it's totally worth it! It's best served with rice or quinoa, cooked as per the packet instructions.

 Portion size: 552g **Kcals:** 612 **Fat:** 18.4g **Saturated fat:** 5.9g **Carbs:** 69g **Sugar:** 24g **Fibre:** 13.5g **Protein:** 35g
Salt: 1.5g **Allergens:** Celery, may contain soya, may contain sulphites

WHAT TO DO

1 Sprinkle the lamb pieces with salt and pepper, then place in a ziplock bag with all the spices and toss gently until covered.

2 Heat the oil in a large heavy-based saucepan set over a medium–high heat. Place the meat in the hot oil and cook for about 4 minutes on each side, until browned. Remove and set aside in a bowl.

3 Reduce the heat to medium–low. Add the celery to the pan and cook gently for 2–3 minutes before adding the carrots. Cook gently for about 10 minutes more, until soft. Add the meat back in, followed by the stock, chopped tomatoes, chickpeas, tomato purée, olives and raisins. Bring to the boil, then reduce the heat and cook on low for about 2 hours. Alternatively, add all the ingredients except the wild rice or quinoa, spring onions, fresh coriander and lemon juice to a slow cooker and cook for 8 hours on a medium setting.

4 When the tagine is nearly ready, cook the wild rice or quinoa as per the packet instructions.

5 When the lamb is done, divide the tagine between four bowls and squeeze over the lemon juice. Garnish with the green part of the spring onions and the fresh coriander. Serve with the cooked wild rice or quinoa.

INGREDIENTS

300g stewing lamb, cut into 2.5cm cubes
salt and freshly ground black pepper
2 tsp ground cumin
1 tsp smoked paprika
1 tsp ground coriander
1 tsp ground cinnamon
1 tsp ground ginger
½ tsp ground turmeric
1 tbsp garlic-infused olive oil
30g/½ stick celery, finely chopped
360g/3 large carrots, finely chopped
500ml homemade low FODMAP chicken stock (page 118) or vegetable stock (page 119)
1 x 400g tin of chopped tomatoes
120g canned chickpeas, drained and rinsed
2 tbsp tomato purée
50g pitted olives, halved
4 tbsp raisins
240g wild rice or quinoa
1 tbsp lemon juice
20g/4 spring onions (green part only), finely sliced
handful of fresh coriander, chopped

Preparation time: 20 minutes
Cooking time: 2½ hours (or 8 hours in a slow cooker)
Serves: 4

Spicy Lamb Cutlets with Cherry Tomato Salsa

Barbecue the cutlets to really bring out the lamb's sweetness and the spicy aromas of the homemade spice mix. For best results, let the lamb rest for a while once cooked – this gives a moister and more tender meat. Serve with fresh coriander sprinkled over your potatoes for an extra twist.

 Portion size: 297g **Kcals:** 556 **Fat:** 35g **Saturated fat:** 14g **Carbs:** 2g **Sugar:** 1.8g **Fibre:** 1.3g **Protein:** 58g **Salt:** 0.7g **Allergens:** None

INGREDIENTS

3 tbsp olive oil
120g/12 lamb cutlets, well trimmed

For the spice mix:
2 tsp paprika
1 tsp ground cumin
1 tsp ground coriander
salt and freshly ground black pepper

For the tomato salsa:
150g/½ cucumber, chopped
120g/10 cherry tomatoes, chopped
50g/10 spring onions (green part only), finely chopped
1 chilli, deseeded and finely chopped
juice of 1 lemon
3 tbsp garlic-infused olive oil
2 tbsp chopped fresh coriander

To serve:
boiled new potatoes
chopped fresh coriander

WHAT TO DO

1 Preheat the grill or a barbecue to 170°C.
2 Mix all the salsa ingredients and a pinch of salt and pepper together in a large bowl. Set aside to let the flavours infuse.
3 Combine all the spice mix ingredients and tip out into a shallow bowl or plate. Drizzle the olive oil over the lamb cutlets, then dip each cutlet in the spice mix and shake off the excess.
4 Grill or barbecue the cutlets for 3–4 minutes on each side.
5 Serve the cutlets with a side of salsa and boiled new potatoes garnished with chopped fresh coriander.

Preparation time: 15 minutes
Cooking time: 10 minutes
Serves: 6

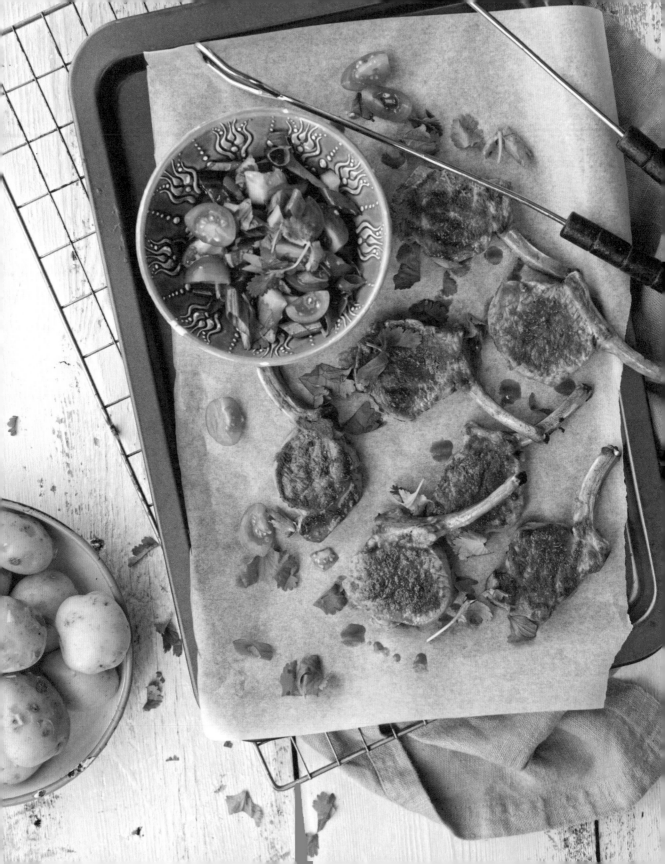

Seekh Kebabs with Crunchy Radish and Tomato Salad

A popular Middle Eastern dish. The accompanying salad perfectly complements and balances this simple-to-cook dish.

 Portion size: 353g **Kcals:** 411 **Fat:** 6.7g **Saturated fat:** 2.8g **Carbs:** 53g **Sugar:** 3.6g **Fibre:** 2.8g **Protein:** 33g **Salt:** 0.3g **Allergens:** None

INGREDIENTS

500g minced beef or lamb
20g/4 spring onions (green part only), finely chopped
1 small green chilli, deseeded and finely chopped (if tolerated)
2cm piece of fresh ginger, peeled and grated
1 tsp garam masala
1 tsp paprika
salt and freshly ground black pepper
lime wedges, to serve
50g Greek yogurt, to serve

For the salad:
300g/½ cucumber, chopped into cubes
260g/2 ripe tomatoes, chopped
34g/5 radishes, quartered
4g/1 handful of fresh coriander, roughly chopped
1 tbsp freshly squeezed lime juice
½ tsp caster sugar or maple syrup

WHAT TO DO

1 Put the mince in a large bowl and add the chopped spring onions, chilli (if using), ginger, garam masala, paprika, salt and pepper and mix well. Set aside to let the spices infuse the meat for at least 20 minutes, but all day is fine too.

2 Place all the salad ingredients in a large bowl and toss together. Cover the bowl with cling film and refrigerate until required. Taste and adjust the seasoning before serving.

3 Preheat the grill to high and lightly grease the grill rack. Soak 12 wooden skewers in cold water for 15 minutes.

4 Divide the meat mixture into 12 equal oval-shaped portions. Wet your hands and shape each portion around a skewer, smoothing over the seam.

5 Place the skewers under the grill and cook for 10–15 minutes, turning occasionally, until the meat is cooked through.

6 Serve the hot kebabs with the chilled salad, lime wedges and a small bowl of Greek yogurt on the side.

Preparation time: 20 minutes
Cooking time: 20 minutes (excluding marinating)
Serves: 4

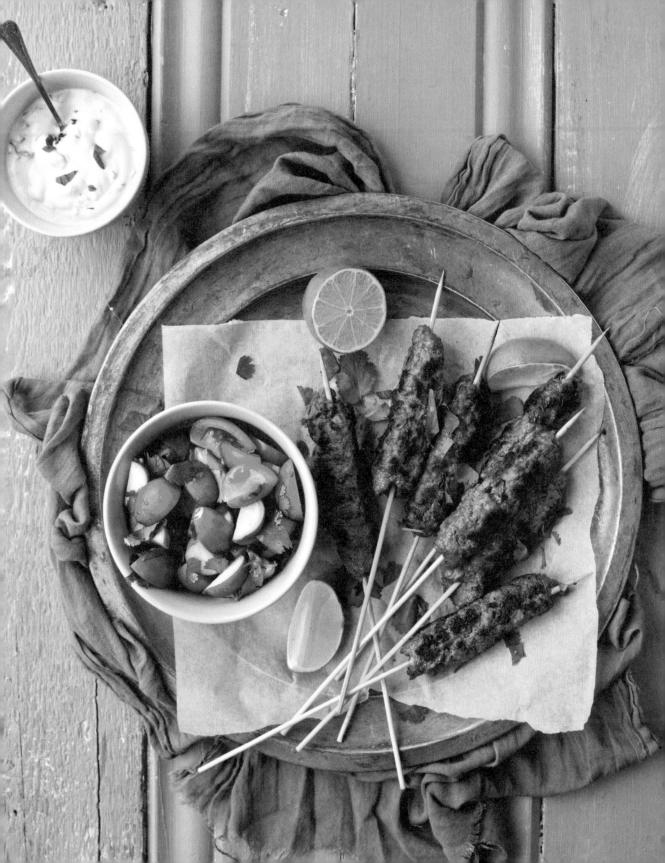

Beef and Bok Choy Stir-Fry

This dish is so simple and beats a takeaway any day. It's the perfect dish when you want something fast after a long day at work. It also works well with prawns.

   Portion size: 340g **Kcals:** 475 **Fat:** 14.3g **Saturated fat:** 3.5g **Carbs:** 44g **Sugar:** 5.7g **Fibre:** 7.4g
Protein: 39g **Salt:** 2.6g **Allergens:** Gluten, sesame, soya, molluscs, may contain eggs, may contain fish

INGREDIENTS

500g lean stir-fry beef, such as sirloin, thinly sliced

½ red chilli, deseeded and finely chopped (optional)

1 tbsp oyster sauce

2 tsp sesame oil

juice of 1 lime, plus lime wedges to serve

1 tbsp garlic-infused rapeseed oil

4cm piece of fresh ginger, peeled and minced

pinch of asafoetida powder

134g/2 medium carrots, thinly sliced lengthways

200g bok choy, sliced

160g/1 red pepper, sliced

15g/3 spring onions (green part only), chopped

2 tbsp low-sodium soya sauce

freshly ground black pepper

200g rice noodles

1 tbsp sesame seeds

1 tsp rapeseed oil

handful of fresh basil leaves, chopped

WHAT TO DO

1 Put the beef in a bowl with the chilli (if using), oyster sauce, sesame oil and half of the lime juice (this can be done in advance for extra marinating time).

2 Heat the garlic-infused oil in a wok set over a high heat. Add the ginger and asafoetida powder and cook for 1 minute. Add the carrots and stir-fry for 2–3 minutes. Add the bok choy and red pepper and cook for 1 minute, followed by the spring onions ,and cook for 1–2 minutes more. Add the soya sauce and a pinch of black pepper and transfer to a large bowl.

3 Cook the noodles as per the packet instructions, then drain.

4 In a separate dry pan, toast the sesame seeds over a medium–low heat, stirring occasionally, for 2–3 minutes, until the seeds turn brown (don't add any oil to the seeds!). The slower the cooking, the nuttier the flavour! Tip out into a bowl or plate.

5 Add the teaspoon of rapeseed oil to the wok and return to a high heat. Add the beef mix and cook for 1–2 minutes, until the beef turns pink, or as per your liking. Add the rest of the lime juice to the beef and swirl it around in the wok for 1 minute before adding the fresh basil. Stir in the cooked vegetables and noodles and toss to combine.

6 Serve the stir-fry sprinkled with the toasted sesame seeds and lime wedges on the side.

Preparation time: 15 minutes
Cooking time: 10 minutes
Serves: 4

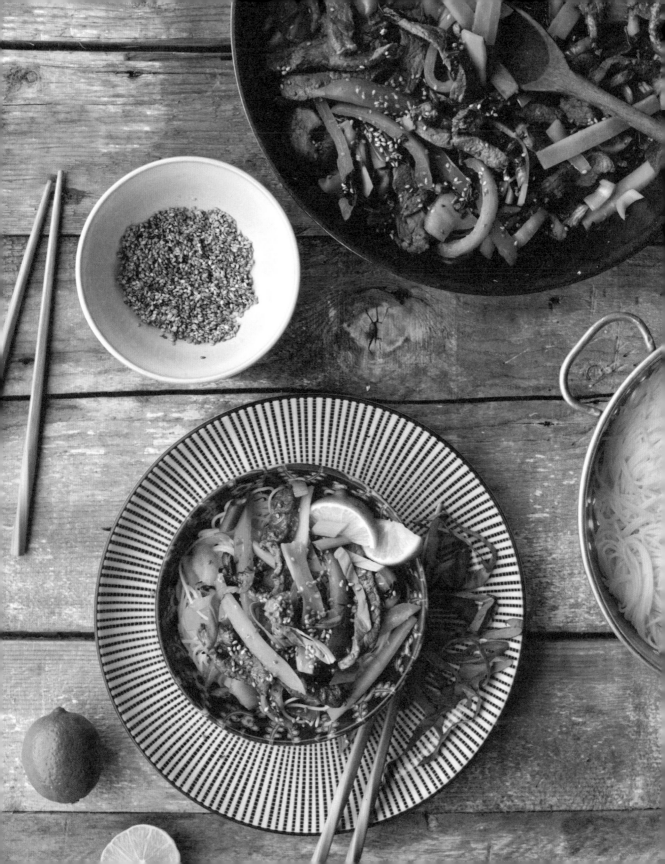

Mediterranean Meatballs

Your family or friends will thank you for cooking these! Super easy and delicious, the meatballs freeze well, so make double for later use. **Remember to keep to the allowed portion of celery (½ celery stick or <30g per serving).**

Portion size: 505g **Kcals:** 580 **Fat:** 15.2g **Saturated fat:** 4.6g **Carbs:** 61g **Sugar:** 14.2g **Fibre:** 12.8g **Protein:** 41g **Salt:** 0.5g **Allergens:** Celery, milk, sulphites, may contain soya, may contain gluten if served with spelt bread

INGREDIENTS

320g gluten-free whole wheat
    spaghetti
450g minced beef or pork
10g/2 spring onions (green part only),
    finely chopped
1 tbsp chopped fresh basil
1 tsp ground cinnamon
1 tbsp garlic-infused olive oil, for
    brushing
4 tsp grated Parmesan, to serve
100% sourdough spelt bread, to serve
    (optional)

For the tomato sauce:

1 tbsp garlic-infused olive oil
60g/1 celery stalk, finely chopped
2 tbsp tomato purée
2 x 400g tins of chopped tomatoes
1 cinnamon stick or ½ tsp ground
    cinnamon
125ml red wine
100ml homemade low FODMAP chicken
    stock (page 118)
salt and freshly ground black pepper

Preparation time: 20 minutes
Cooking time: 1 hour
Serves: 4

WHAT TO DO

1 For the tomato sauce, heat the oil in a large pan set over a low heat. Add the celery and fry for 1–2 minutes. Add the tomato purée and cook for a few minutes, followed by the canned tomatoes, cinnamon, red wine and stock. Season to taste. Bring to the boil, then turn the heat down very low and simmer for 1 hour, stirring occasionally.

2 Preheat the grill to its highest setting.

3 When the sauce is almost ready, start cooking the spaghetti as per the packet instructions.

4 For the meatballs, place the mince, spring onions, basil and cinnamon in a bowl. Season with freshly ground black pepper and mix well.

5 Roll small amounts of the mince mixture into balls. You should make 12–16 meatballs. Brush the meatballs with a little oil and place on a baking tray. Place under the grill to cook for 8–10 minutes, turning occasionally and brushing them with a little more oil as they brown.

6 To serve, stir the cooked spaghetti through the sauce. Divide between four plates and serve with three or four meatballs on top, then sprinkle with Parmesan cheese. Serve with some 100% sourdough spelt bread on the side if you need a carbo-hydrate boost pre-competition or post-training.

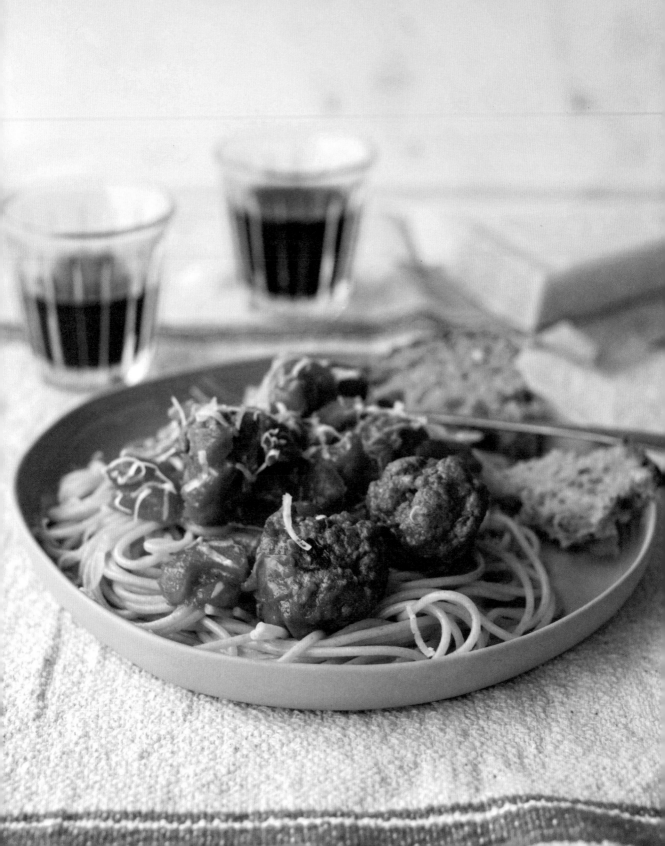

Fillet Steak with Slow-Cooked Tomatoes, Salsa Verde and Watercress

The fillet is probably the nicest and most expensive cut of beef. It's very lean and tender due to the short fibres in the meat. Salsa verde not only contains lots of vitamins, it also bursts with freshness from the herbs and savoury anchovies. With the slow-cooked tomatoes and watercress salad, this is a recipe that will have you looking forward to steak night. **Remember to stick to no more than 1 tablespoon of balsamic vinegar per sitting.**

Portion size: 308g **Kcals:** 519 **Fat:** 45g **Saturated fat:** 8.3g **Carbs:** 4.8g **Sugar:** 4.3g **Fibre:** 2.5g **Protein:** 23g **Salt:** 1.5g
Allergens: Mustard, fish, sulphites

INGREDIENTS

4 x 100g fillet steaks

For the slow-cooked tomatoes:

520g/4 vine-ripened tomatoes or 16
    cherry tomatoes
2 sprigs of fresh thyme
splash of balsamic vinegar
splash of olive oil
pinch of caster sugar
salt and freshly ground black pepper

For the salsa verde:

2 tsp white wine vinegar
4–5 fresh basil sprigs, leaves only
handful of fresh flat-leaf parsley
6g/2 tinned anchovy fillets, drained
    and finely chopped
3 tsp capers
100ml garlic-infused olive oil

For the watercress salad:

100g watercress
4 tbsp olive oil
1 tsp white wine vinegar
1 tsp Dijon mustard
pinch of salt

WHAT TO DO

1 Preheat the oven to 120°C.

2 To prepare the slow-cooked tomatoes, combine the thyme, vinegar, oil, sugar and seasoning and dip the tomatoes (still on the vine) into the mix, coating them completely. Place on a baking tray and gently roast them in the oven for 15–20 minutes.

3 Heat a large frying pan over a high heat until it's smoking hot, then brush with olive oil.

4 Season one side of the steak and put it in the hot pan, seasoned side down. Cook for 1–2 minutes, until nicely browned. Just before turning it over, season the raw side and brown for 1–2 minutes more. Turn down the heat and cook to your liking. This can take another minute on each side for rare, 2–3 minutes for medium and 4–5 minutes for well done.

5 To make the salsa verde, pour the vinegar into a blender with the basil leaves, parsley, anchovies and capers and blend to a purée. With the motor still running, gradually add just enough of the olive oil to give a sauce-like consistency.

6 To make the watercress salad, simply toss all the ingredients together and season to taste.

7 To serve the steaks, place the slow-cooked tomatoes on the side and spoon the salsa verde over the steak. Add the watercress salad on the side.

Preparation time: 15 minutes
Cooking time: 25 minutes
Serves: 4

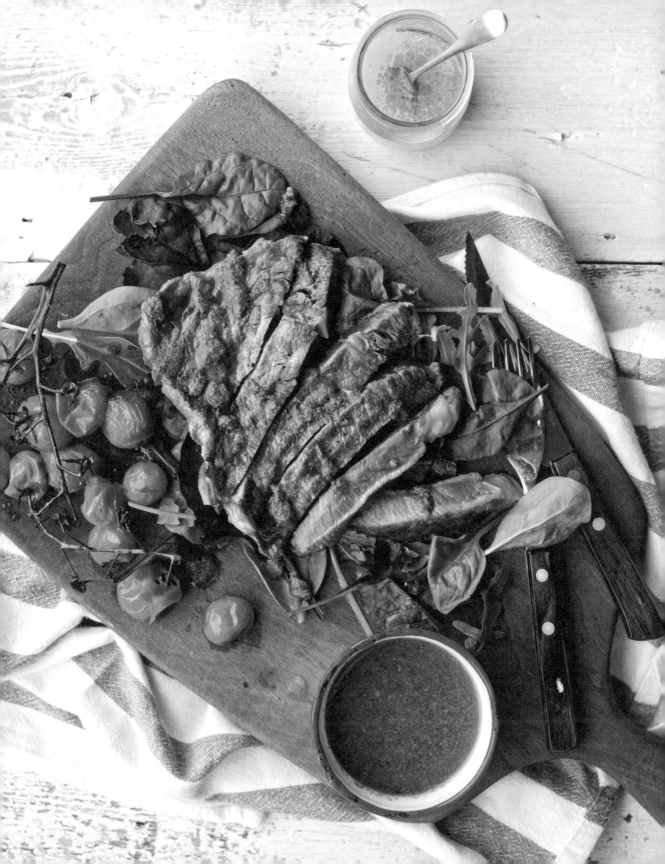

Salmon Fish Cakes with Spinach and Strawberry Salad

This fish cake and salad combo is delicious and satisfying. If you like, you can substitute the salmon for other fish, such as tuna, crab or haddock. **Remember to use a maximum of 1 tablespoon of balsamic vinegar per serving. And as always, don't forget that only the green part of spring onions is allowed on a low FODMAP diet!**

Portion size: 407g **Kcals:** 514 **Fat:** 26.7g **Saturated fat:** 4.5g **Carbs:** 31g **Sugar:** 6.4g **Fibre:** 6g **Protein:** 34g
Salt: 1.5g **Allergens:** Milk, fish, mustard, eggs, may contain soya, may contain sulphites, may contain lupin

INGREDIENTS

300g potatoes, peeled and cut into chunks
400g fresh or tinned salmon
1 tsp olive oil
20g/4 spring onions (green part only), finely chopped
100ml lactose-free milk
salt and freshly ground black pepper
juice of 1 lemon
½ bunch of fresh chives

For the crumb coating:
50g/2 small slices of whole wheat or
    multigrain gluten-free bread
handful of chopped fresh parsley
1 heaped tbsp cornflour
2 eggs, beaten
1 tsp rapeseed oil

For the salad:
200g baby spinach
160g rocket
160g strawberries, halved
2 tbsp pumpkin seeds

For the dressing:
3 tbsp olive oil
1 tbsp balsamic vinegar
1 tsp wholegrain mustard
1 tsp maple syrup
1 tsp lemon juice

To serve: fresh coriander leaves, lemon wedges,
sweet chilli sauce (page 134)

WHAT TO DO

1 Boil the potatoes for about 15 minutes, until just soft. Drain and let them steam dry.

2 If using tinned fish, drain it well.

3 Heat the oil in a pan set over a medium heat, then add the spring onions and milk and cook for 3 minutes. Season well, then add the lemon juice and chives. Add the warm milk mixture to the potatoes and mash well, then stir in the fish.

4 To coat the cakes, place the bread in a food processor and blitz into breadcrumbs. Tip into a shallow dish and stir in the parsley. Place the cornflour and beaten eggs in two separate shallow dishes.

5 Shape the fish into approximately 16 mini fish cakes. Dredge them in the cornflour and shake off the excess, then dip in the beaten egg before pressing gently into the breadcrumbs. Chill in the fridge for at least 30 minutes before cooking.

6 Heat the teaspoon of rapeseed oil in a frying pan set over a medium heat. Fry the fish cakes for 5 minutes on each side, until they turn crisp and golden.

7 Create the salad by combining the spinach, rocket, strawberries and pumpkin seeds. Whisk all the dressing ingredients together, then pour it over the salad and toss to combine. Season with black pepper.

8 Scatter the warm fish cakes with fresh coriander leaves and serve the salad, lemon wedges and sweet chilli sauce on the side.

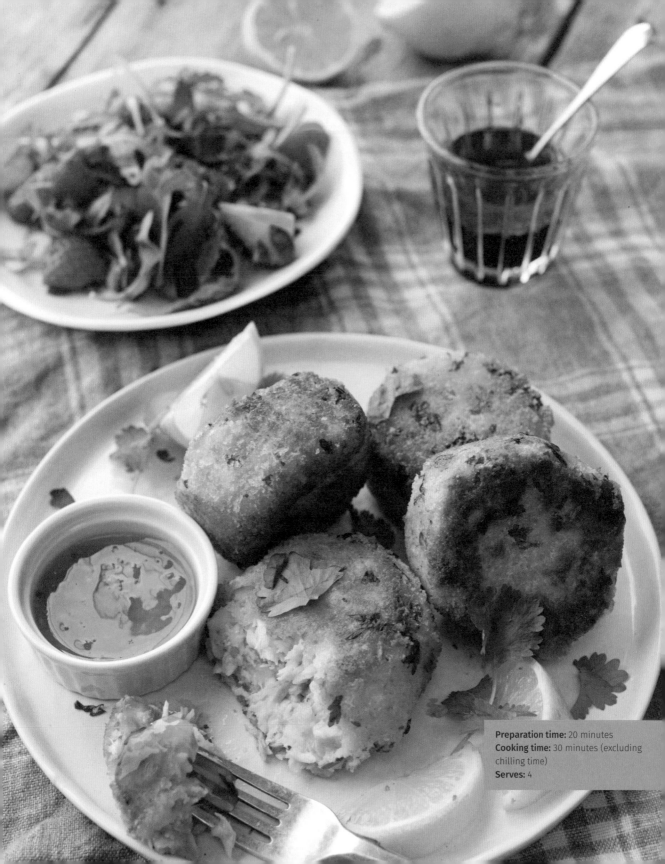

Preparation time: 20 minutes
Cooking time: 30 minutes (excluding chilling time)
Serves: 4

Warm Steak Salad with Tomato, Cucumber and Basil

This is a quick and easy salad that is simply delicious and bursting with summer flavours. The cast iron grill gives the steak a mouth-watering finish. It's the perfect meal for a summer evening when you want something lighter on the stomach, plus it's a good way to use up any leftovers.

 Portion size: 243g **Kcals:** 265 **Fat:** 15.7g **Saturated fat:** 3.6g **Carbs:** 5.4g **Sugar:** 4.8g **Fibre:** 1.1g **Protein:** 25g
Salt: 1.4g **Allergens:** Gluten, sesame, soya, may contain fish

INGREDIENTS

400g sirloin or striploin steak

For the marinade:

1 tbsp fish or soya sauce
1 tbsp lemon or lime juice
1 tsp caster sugar
1 tsp ground black pepper
1 tsp sesame oil

For the salad:

300g/1 cucumber, deseeded and
    sliced
144g/12 cherry tomatoes, halved
3–4 tbsp garlic-infused olive oil
1 tbsp fish or soya sauce
handful of fresh basil leaves, chopped
juice of ½ lemon

To serve:

660g/4 baked potatoes (see page 42)

WHAT TO DO

1 Mix all the marinade ingredients together. Pour it over the steaks and leave for 20 minutes.

2 Heat a cast iron grill pan until it's smoking hot. Add the steaks and cook for 2–3 minutes on each side for rare, 3–4 minutes for medium and 5–6 minutes for well done. Allow the steaks to rest for a few minutes before slicing.

3 To make the salad, simply toss all the salad ingredients together in a large bowl.

4 Serve the steaks with the salad and a baked potato.

Preparation time: 20 minutes
Cooking time: 6–12 minutes
Serves: 4

Baked Hake with Homemade Tartar Sauce

This is a light and fragrant dish. You can use any white fish for this recipe. **Serve with broccoli, but stick to the recommended portion size (<47g/2 tablespoons) to keep within the low FODMAP advice. Also remember to keep to one-quarter of the tartar sauce if made with Greek yogurt.**

  Portion size: 364g **Kcals:** 326 **Fat:** 6.9g **Saturated fat:** 1.8g **Carbs:** 24g **Sugar:** 5.6g **Fibre:** 6.1g **Protein:** 39g **Salt:** 0.8g **Allergens:** Mustard, fish, eggs, sulphites, milk, may contain soya, may contain lupin, may contain gluten if spelt bread is used

WHAT TO DO

1 Preheat the oven to 200°C. Line a large baking tray with tin foil and brush with a little oil.
2 To make the tartar sauce, mix together the yogurt, lemon juice, mustard, parsley and black pepper in a small bowl. Chill until ready to serve.
3 Meanwhile, place the bread in a food processor and blitz into breadcrumbs. Tip into a shallow bowl and stir in the grated Parmesan and parsley.
4 Place the flour and beaten egg in separate shallow bowls.
5 Season the hake with freshly ground black pepper. Working with one piece at a time, dip the hake first into the flour, shaking off the excess, then into the egg and finally into the breadcrumbs. Place on the prepared baking tray and bake in the oven for 15 minutes, until cooked through.
6 Meanwhile, steam the green beans and broccoli.
7 Serve the baked hake with the steamed vegetables and tartar sauce.

INGREDIENTS

olive oil, for brushing
75g/2 medium slices of gluten-free or 100% sourdough spelt bread
1 tbsp grated Parmesan
1 tbsp chopped fresh parsley
40g gluten-free plain flour
1 egg, lightly beaten
600g/4 hake fillets (approx. 150g each)
320g green beans
180g/4 broccoli florets

For the tartar sauce:
150g low-fat Greek yogurt or cow's milk natural yogurt
1 tbsp freshly squeezed lemon juice
1 tsp Dijon mustard
handful of fresh parsley, chopped, to garnish
freshly ground black pepper

Preparation time: 15 minutes
Cooking time: 15 minutes
Serves: 4

Prawn Risotto with Asparagus

This risotto is light yet creamy. **Make sure you use FODMAP-friendly stock and keep to the recommended portion size of asparagus (1 spear per serving) and celery (½ stick per serving).**

 Portion size: 560g **Kcals:** 450 **Fat:** 15.8g **Saturated fat:** 5.7g **Carbs:** 40g **Sugar:** 1g **Fibre:** 1.5g **Protein:** 27g
Salt: 2g **Allergens:** Celery, crustaceans, milk, sulphites

INGREDIENTS

600ml homemade low FODMAP
    chicken stock (page 118)
1 tbsp butter
2 tsp garlic-infused oil
pinch of asafoetida powder
60g/1 celery stick, finely diced
100g Arborio rice
100ml dry white wine
200g large cooked peeled prawns
20g/2 asparagus spears, steamed
    and diced
1 tbsp grated lemon zest
1 tbsp chopped fresh chives
freshly ground black pepper

WHAT TO DO

1 Place the stock in a saucepan and keep on a low heat while you cook the risotto.
2 Heat the butter and garlic-infused oil in a separate large saucepan set over a low heat. Add the asafoetida powder, followed by the diced celery, and cook slowly for about 5 minutes, until soft.
3 Add the rice and raise the heat to medium. Stir for 1–2 minutes, until the grains look toasted but not browned. Add the wine and stir until it has been absorbed into the rice, then start adding the stock one ladle at a time, stirring frequently. Wait until it has all been absorbed into the rice before adding the next ladleful of stock. It should take 15–20 minutes to cook the rice. The ideal risotto is soft but still has a bite. Use extra boiling water if you run out of stock.
4 Five minutes before you feel it's cooked, stir in the prawns, asparagus and lemon zest and continue to cook for 5 minutes, stirring gently.
5 Remove from the heat when the risotto is done and stir in the chives and a pinch of freshly ground black pepper. Serve straight away.

Preparation time: 15 minutes
Cooking time: 20 minutes
Serves: 2

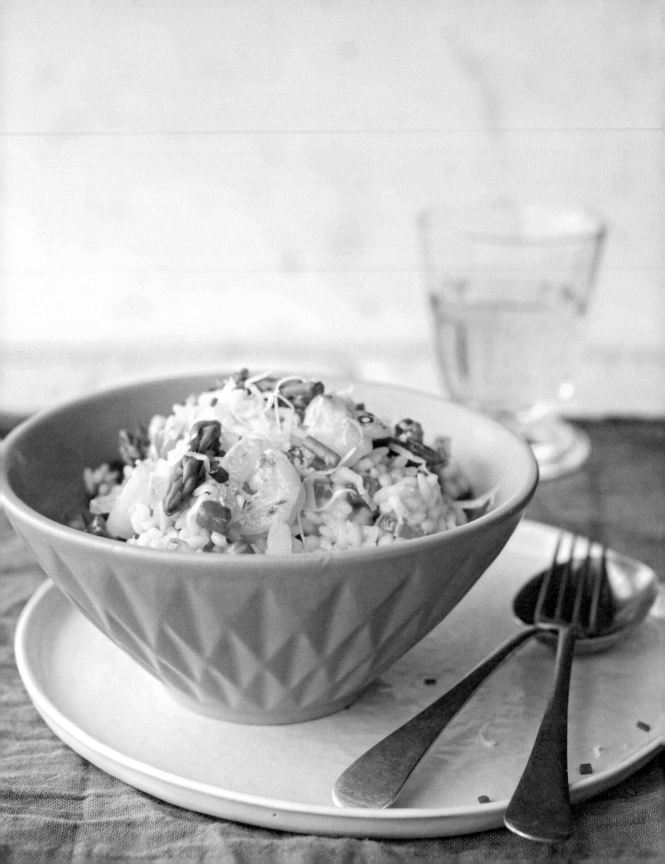

Cajun Spiced Salmon

Salmon is an oily fish containing high-quality protein, vitamin D and omega-3 fatty acids. The coriander seeds give the dish a lemony, citrus flavour when crushed due to the presence of terpenes. It's recommended to eat at least one serving of oily fish each week for general health.

Portion size: 498g **Kcals:** 500 **Fat:** 34g **Saturated fat:** 6.4g **Carbs:** 11.6g **Sugar:** 7.3g **Fibre:** 5.1g **Protein:** 36.3g **Salt:** 4.5g **Allergens:** Fish

INGREDIENTS

2 x 150g salmon fillets, skin on
2 tbsp olive oil
2 tbsp Cajun spice (or less if you like)
260g/2 ripe plum tomatoes, diced finely
20g/4 spring onions (green part only), sliced
handful of fresh coriander leaves and fresh basil leaves
1 tsp crushed coriander seeds
juice of 1 lemon
salt and freshly ground black pepper
100g baby spinach
40g rocket
30g bean sprouts, to garnish (optional)
lemon wedges, to serve

WHAT TO DO

1 Brush the salmon fillets with a little of the olive oil and sprinkle them with the Cajun spice. Set aside.
2 To make the dressing, combine the diced tomatoes, spring onions, fresh herbs and crushed coriander seeds with the remaining olive oil, half the lemon juice and some salt and pepper in a bowl. Set aside.
3 Heat a non-stick frying pan set over a medium heat. Add the salmon and cook for about 4 minutes on each side, taking care not to burn the spices. Transfer to a plate.
4 While the salmon is resting, wilt down the spinach in a separate hot pan with the remaining lemon juice.
5 Place the salmon on a bed of spinach and rocket. Spoon over the tomato dressing and garnish with the bean sprouts, if using. Serve with lemon wedges on the side.

Preparation time: 10 minutes
Cooking time: 15 minutes
Serves: 2

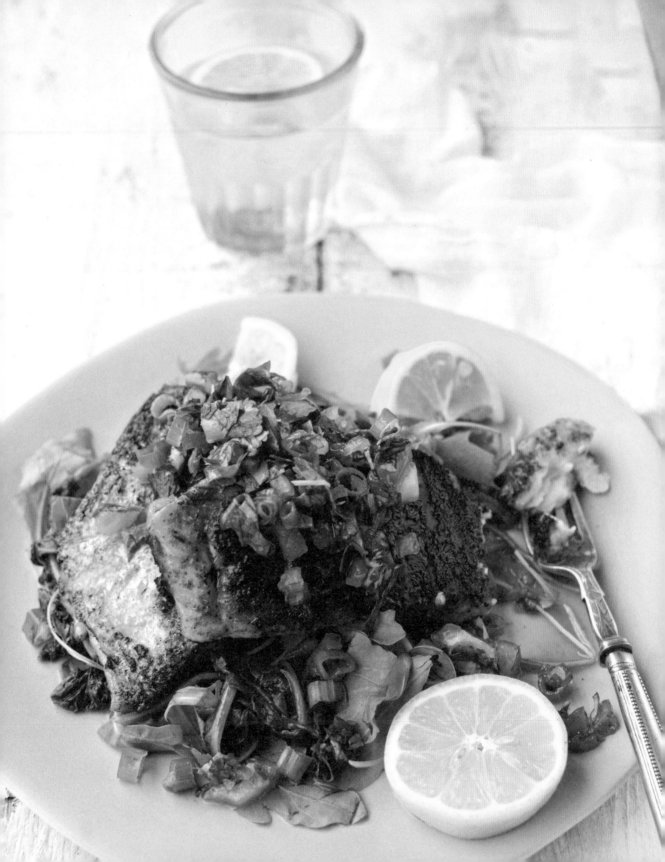

Mild Monkfish Curry with Prawns and Coconut Milk

Monkfish has a mild, sweet taste and a texture similar to lobster. In fact, it's sometimes called 'poor man's lobster'. Combined with the fresh prawns and creamy **coconut milk (for low FODMAP, limit your portion to 125ml)**, this seafood medley is packed with protein and goodness.

 Portion size: 557g **Kcals:** 599 **Fat:** 28.1g **Saturated fat:** 20.1g **Carbs:** 49g **Sugar:** 4g **Fibre:** 4.2g **Protein:** 31g **Salt:** 0.6g **Allergens:** Fish, crustaceans, tree nuts

INGREDIENTS

2 tbsp rapeseed oil
160g/1 green pepper, thinly sliced
160g/1 red pepper, thinly sliced
80g green beans, chopped into thirds
60g/12 spring onions (green part only), chopped
1 dessertspoon red curry paste (page 134)
750ml coconut milk (approx. 2 tins)
6 x 150g pieces of monkfish
200g fresh prawns
960g cooked basmati rice (160g per person), to serve
3 tbsp flaked almonds, to garnish
green salad, to serve (optional)

WHAT TO DO

1 Heat the rapeseed oil in a deep, wide-based pan set over a high heat. Quickly fry the vegetables until they are just beginning to soften. Add the red curry paste and cook for a further 2–3 minutes, until the vegetables are fully coated with the paste.

2 Pour the coconut milk into the pan and bring to the boil, then reduce the heat and nestle the monkfish and prawns into the sauce. Cover and simmer gently for 8–10 minutes, until the fish is cooked through. Baste the monkfish with the sauce now and then as it cooks. If the sauce is too thick, add some extra water or even white wine if you're feeling indulgent and bring to the boil before serving.

3 Remove the monkfish from the pan and place on top of a bed of boiled basmati rice. Divide the curry sauce and prawns between the plates, **making sure to take just 125ml if you're following the low FODMAP diet.** Serve scattered with a couple of flaked almonds and a green salad.

Preparation time: 10 minutes
Cooking time: 25 minutes
Serves: 6

Peri-Peri Chicken with Cider

No need for fast food when you have this recipe in your back pocket. The spice mix provides a range of healthy and yummy flavours. For best results, let the chicken rest in the spice mix overnight. Adding the cider of your choice makes this recipe unique to you and gives the chicken a spicy glaze with hints of apple sweetness.

  Portion size: 172g **Kcals:** 150 **Fat:** 1.3g **Saturated fat:** 0.4g **Carbs:** 2.2g **Sugar:** 2.2g **Fibre:** 0.5g **Protein:** 29g
Salt: 1g **Allergens:** Sulphites, may contain gluten

WHAT TO DO

1 Preheat the oven to 190°C.
2 Combine all the spices and salt in a bowl and mix well. Put the chicken pieces into a large freezer bag and add in the spice mix. Seal the bag and shake well to make sure all the chicken is coated.
3 Place the chicken on a baking dish, drizzle with the oil and cook in the oven for 10–15 minutes. Remove from the oven and pour the cider on top of the chicken. Return to the oven and cook for a further 25–30 minutes, basting regularly, until the chicken is coated with a nice spicy glaze.
4 Serve with a large salad and wild rice (not included in the nutritional analysis).

INGREDIENTS

2 tsp chilli powder
1 tsp paprika
1 tsp ground cumin
1 tsp rock salt
½ tsp ground coriander
½ tsp dried oregano
6 x 120g chicken breasts, diced
3 tbsp garlic-infused oil
300ml your favourite cider
green salad, to serve (optional)
steamed wild rice, to serve (optional)

Preparation time: 10 minutes
Cooking time: 45 minutes
Serves: 6

Mexican Chicken Fajitas

This colourful, satisfying Mexican favourite never disappoints and is great for feeding a group, no matter what age. Corn and gluten-free tortillas, as alternatives to wheat-based tortillas, are widely available.

   Portion size: 497g **Kcals:** 442 **Fat:** 11.2g **Saturated fat:** 4.4g **Carbs:** 5.9g **Sugar:** 12.8g **Fibre:** 6.3g **Protein:** 34g
Salt: 0.9g **Allergens:** Gluten, milk, may contain soya, may contain sesame

INGREDIENTS

1 tbsp rapeseed oil
pinch of asafoetida powder
430g/4 small chicken breasts, cut into bite-size
   pieces
160g/1 yellow pepper, cut into strips
160g/1 red pepper, cut into strips
160g/1 green pepper, cut into strips

For the spice mix:
2 tsp ground cumin
2 tsp ground coriander
2 tsp smoked paprika
1 tsp dried oregano
½ tsp chilli powder (optional)

For the salsa:
520g/4 ripe plum tomatoes, finely chopped
20g/4 spring onions (green part only), finely sliced
½ fresh chilli, deseeded and chopped (optional)
handful of fresh coriander leaves, chopped
juice of 1 lime
freshly ground black pepper

To serve:
320g/8 mini corn tortillas
100g iceberg lettuce, shredded
40g grated Cheddar
50g Greek yogurt or low-fat sour cream (optional)
lime wedges

WHAT TO DO

1 For the spice mix, combine all the spices together in a small bowl and set aside.

2 To make the salsa, combine all the ingredients in a separate bowl and set aside.

3 Heat the rapeseed oil in a pan set over a medium–high heat. Add the pinch of asafoetida powder and cook for about 30 seconds before adding the chicken pieces. Cook for 3–4 minutes, then add the pepper strips and spice mix and continue cooking for another 3–4 minutes, until the chicken is turning golden brown and is cooked through.

4 Meanwhile, warm the tortillas in the oven or microwave as per the packet instructions.

5 Assemble the fajitas by placing some shredded lettuce, a spoonful of the chicken mix, a spoonful of salsa, a sprinkle of grated cheese and a dollop of yogurt on each warm tortilla. Wrap up tightly and serve with lime wedges on the side.

Preparation time: 30 minutes
Cooking time: 10 minutes
Serves: 4

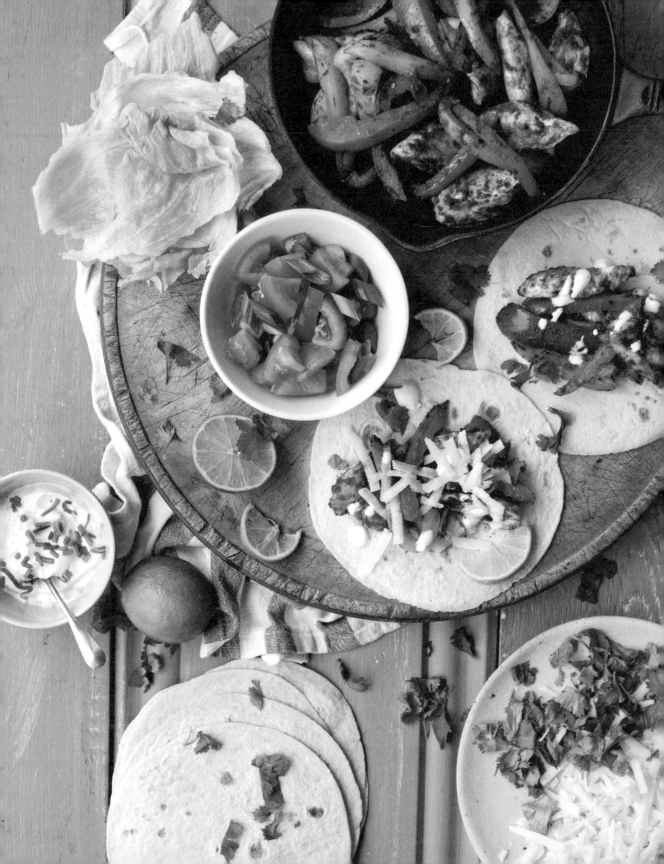

Chicken Skewers with Corn and Rice Salad

This tasty dish is fab on the BBQ or fresh off the grill. It's simple to make, but do give the chicken time to marinate overnight or put it in the fridge in the morning. **Remember, the allowed serving size for sweetcorn is 43g/½ cob per portion.** These skewers also work well with the low FODMAP coleslaw on page 128.

  Portion size: 437g **Kcals:** 493 **Fat:** 9g **Saturated fat:** 1.5g **Carbs:** 63g **Sugar:** 16.7g **Fibre:** 6.1g **Protein:** 37.3g **Salt:** 1.2g **Allergens:** Soya, gluten, sesame, may contain mustard, milk and sulphites if served with the low FODMAP coleslaw

INGREDIENTS

10g/2 spring onions (green part only)
200ml orange juice
2 tbsp maple syrup
zest and juice of 1 lime
2 tbsp low-sodium soya sauce
1 tbsp sesame oil
1 tsp ground cumin
480g/4 chicken breasts, cut into pieces
160g/1 red pepper, cut into chunks
½ courgette, cut into chunks
low FODMAP coleslaw (page 128),
    to serve
lemon wedges, to serve

For the corn and rice salad:
260g brown rice
160g/1 small tin of sweetcorn kernels
150g/12 cherry tomatoes, diced
juice of ½ lemon
1 tbsp olive oil
1 tbsp chopped fresh chives
80g rocket

WHAT TO DO

1 Combine the spring onions, orange juice, maple syrup, lime zest and juice, soya sauce, sesame oil and cumin in a bowl. Add the chicken, cover with cling film and marinate for at least 30 minutes or overnight.

2 Meanwhile, cook the rice as per the packet instructions and set aside to cool.

3 To make the salad, combine the cooled rice, sweetcorn and cherry tomatoes in a bowl. Drizzle with the lemon juice and olive oil, sprinkle with the chives and mix together. Place the rocket leaves around the edges of the bowl. Place in the fridge to chill before serving.

4 Preheat the grill to medium. Soak eight wooden skewers in cold water for 15 minutes.

5 To assemble the skewers, place a piece of chicken on a skewer, followed by a vegetable chunk (either red pepper or courgette). Repeat until all the chicken and veg are used up.

6 Cook the skewers under the grill for about 8 minutes on each side, until the chicken is cooked through and the vegetables are lightly charred.

7 Meanwhile, place the leftover marinade in a small pan, bring to the boil and cook for 2–3 minutes. Drizzle the boiled marinade over the skewers.

8 Serve with the corn and rice salad, low FODMAP coleslaw and some lemon wedges on the side.

Preparation time: 30 minutes (excluding marinating time)
Cooking time: 45 minutes
Serves: 4

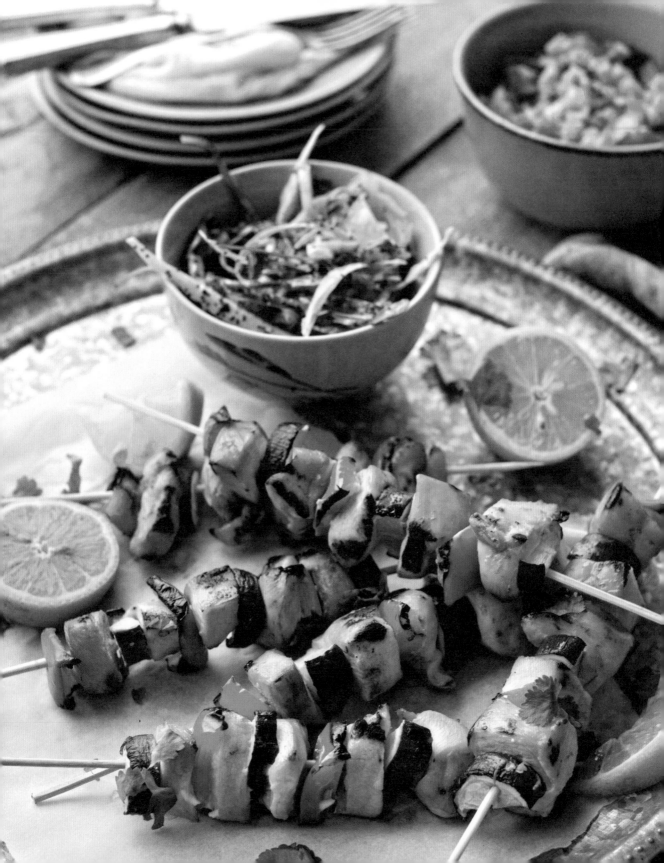

Chicken Tikka Masala

Now said to be the world's most popular Indian dish, tikka masala actually originated from the kitchens of Bangladeshi chefs in the UK! **If you can tolerate it, cream can be used instead of Greek yogurt in this recipe. Just remember to keep to the allowed portion size of normal yogurt (<50g per serving).**

  Portion size: 351g **Kcals:** 446 **Fat:** 8.8g **Saturated fat:** 3.2g **Carbs:** 54g **Sugar:** 4.3g **Fibre:** 2.8g
Protein: 36g **Salt:** 0.3g **Allergens:** Milk

INGREDIENTS

260g brown basmati rice
340g/4 ripe plum tomatoes
150g Greek yogurt
4cm piece of fresh ginger, peeled and grated
1 tbsp garlic-infused rapeseed oil
2 bay leaves
pinch of asafoetida powder
¼ green chilli, deseeded and finely chopped (optional)
1 tsp ground cumin
1 tsp ground coriander
½ tsp paprika
½ tsp garam masala
¼ tsp ground turmeric
pinch of salt
480g/4 medium chicken breasts, cut into pieces
15g/3 spring onions (green part only), finely chopped
125ml water
handful of fresh coriander leaves, chopped

WHAT TO DO

1 Cook the rice as per the packet instructions.
2 Place the tomatoes, yogurt and ginger in a blender and blend until a thick sauce forms, then set aside.
3 Heat the oil in a large saucepan (one with a tight-fitting lid) set over a medium heat. Add the bay leaves and asafoetida powder and cook for 1 minute. Reduce the heat to medium–low and add the chilli (if using), cumin, coriander, paprika, garam masala, turmeric and salt and stir for 1 minute, until you can smell the aroma of the spices. Watch carefully so the spice mixture doesn't burn.
4 Tip in the chicken pieces and fry, stirring occasionally, for 3 minutes. Stir the tomato and yogurt mixture and the spring onions into the pan, cover and reduce to a low heat. Simmer for 5–7 minutes, until the chicken is cooked through.
5 Bring the water to the boil while the chicken mixture is simmering, then add the boiling water to the chicken and simmer for a further 1 minute, stirring, until droplets of oil appear on the surface.
6 Serve hot with the cooked basmati rice and garnish with the chopped fresh coriander.

Preparation time: 15 minutes
Cooking time: 20 minutes
Serves: 4

Chicken Pasta with Low FODMAP Pesto

This is an easy dish with tons of flavour. It's also one of those great dishes if time is not on your side and it shows you how a FODMAP-friendly pesto can be achieved!

 Portion size: 430g **Kcals:** 662 **Fat:** 43g **Saturated fat:** 7.4g **Carbs:** 22.2g **Sugar:** 5.4g **Fibre:** 7.3g **Protein:** 43g **Salt:** 2g
Allergens: Tree nuts, milk, may contain eggs, may contain lupin

WHAT TO DO

1 Cook the pasta as per the packet instructions. Drain well and place in a large bowl.
2 Heat the garlic-infused oil in a frying pan set over a medium heat. Add the chicken and cook for 3–4 minutes, until golden. Add the cherry tomatoes and olives and cook another 2–3 minutes, until the chicken is all cooked through. Take off the heat and season with black pepper.
3 While the chicken is cooking, add the green beans to a saucepan of boiling water and cook for 7–8 minutes, until soft. Drain and add to the chicken.
4 To make the pesto, blend all the ingredients together until smooth. Add more oil if needed until you get the desired creamy consistency.
5 Add the chicken, tomatoes, olives, green beans and pesto to the pasta and mix to combine. Divide the pasta between two plates and season with freshly ground black pepper before serving.

INGREDIENTS

120g whole wheat gluten-free pasta
2 tsp garlic-infused olive oil
240g/2 chicken breasts, cut into pieces
100g/8 cherry tomatoes, halved
60g/12 black olives, rinsed if in brine
freshly ground black pepper
160g green beans, trimmed

For the pesto:
1 large bunch of fresh basil, chopped
juice of 1 lemon
30g grated Parmesan
25g pine nuts
20g almonds
2 tbsp garlic-infused olive oil

Preparation time: 15 minutes
Cooking time: 15 minutes
Serves: 2

Tofu Yellow Curry with Rice

This is the ultimate curry! It's creamy, spicy and fragrant. If you're not vegetarian, swap in your favourite protein. Prawns, chicken and beef would all work perfectly with this dish. The curry paste will keep in the fridge for two weeks.

  Portion size: 482g **Kcals:** 525 **Fat:** 17g **Saturated fat:** 5.7g **Carbs:** 64g **Sugar:** 10.8g **Fibre:** 9.2g **Protein:** 23.7g **Salt:** 1.8g **Allergens:** Fish, celery, sulphites, soya

INGREDIENTS

260g brown basmati rice
2 tsp garlic-infused rapeseed oil
400g extra-firm tofu, drained and
    cut into 2cm cubes
360g/4 carrots, thinly sliced
160g/1 red pepper, thinly sliced
250ml homemade low FODMAP stock (page 118)
200ml light coconut milk
2 handfuls of fresh coriander leaves
10g/2 spring onions (green part only),
    finely chopped

For the yellow curry paste:
15g/3 spring onions (green part only), thinly sliced
1 stalk of lemongrass, outer layer removed
3 tbsp light coconut milk
2 tbsp tomato purée
juice of 1 lime
1 tbsp chopped fresh ginger
4 tsp Thai fish sauce (or soya sauce if vegetarian)
2 tsp chopped fresh coriander (leaves and stalks)
1–2 tsp paprika depending on how hot you like it!
1 tsp ground turmeric
1 tsp ground cumin
1 tsp ground coriander
1 tsp garlic-infused oil
½ tsp black peppercorns
¼ tsp ground cinnamon

WHAT TO DO

1 Put all the yellow curry paste ingredients in a blender and blitz until smooth. Add a little bit more coconut milk if it's too thick.
2 Cook the rice according to the packet instructions.
3 Meanwhile, heat 1 teaspoon of the garlic-infused rapeseed oil in a large non-stick pan set over a medium heat. Add the curry paste and cook for 1–2 minutes. Add the tofu and cook, tossing occasionally, for 4–5 minutes, until golden. Transfer to a plate.
4 Heat the remaining teaspoon of oil in the pan and reduce the heat to medium–low. Add the carrots and red pepper and cook for 5–7 minutes, stirring occasionally, until the vegetables begin to soften.
5 Add the stock and coconut milk to the pan and bring up to a simmer. Add the tofu back in and continue to cook for 8–10 minutes, stirring occasionally, until the vegetables are tender.
6 Sprinkle with the coriander leaves and spring onions and serve with the rice.

Preparation time: 20 minutes
Cooking time: 25 minutes
Serves: 4

Stir-Fried Tofu with Chilli and Lime

Tofu originated in China and the story goes that a Chinese cook created it 2,000 years ago when he accidently curdled soy milk when he added nigari seaweed to it. Either way, it makes for a great vegetarian dish, but you can substitute chicken if you prefer. **Remember, the allowed serving size for sweetcorn is 43g per sitting.**

   Portion size: 373g **Kcals:** 429 **Fat:** 16.6g **Saturated fat:** 2.6g **Carbs:** 47g **Sugar:** 19.8g **Fibre:** 8.3g
Protein: 18.3g **Salt:** 1.5g **Allergens:** Gluten, peanuts, soya, sulphites, may contain milk

WHAT TO DO

1 Mix the sweet chilli sauce, soya sauce and lime juice in a jug. Place the tofu in a bowl and pour over half of the sauce. Set aside to marinate for 20 minutes.
2 Heat 1 tablespoon of the oil in a wok set over a high heat. Add the tofu and stir-fry until it's browned all over. Set aside and keep warm.
3 Clean out the wok and add the remaining tablespoon of oil. Stir-fry the carrots, green beans, spring onions and baby corn over a high heat until just tender. Stir in the remaining sauce and the cooked rice noodles, then gently stir in the cooked tofu. Scatter over the peanuts and coriander and serve immediately.

INGREDIENTS

100ml sweet chilli sauce (page 134)
2 tbsp dark soya sauce
2 tbsp lime juice
250g firm tofu, cut into cubes
2 tbsp garlic-infused olive oil
180g/2 carrots, peeled into ribbons
250g green beans, chopped
30g/6 spring onions (green part only), sliced diagonally
100g baby corn cobs, sliced diagonally
450g cooked rice noodles
50g dry roasted peanuts, chopped
2 tbsp chopped fresh coriander

Preparation time: 20 minutes
Cooking time: 20 minutes
Serves: 4

Mini Egg Frittatas with Parsnip Chips

These mini frittatas can be eaten hot or cold. Although they're included in the dinner chapter, they are also appropriate for breakfast, lunch or as a snack!

 Portion size: 289g **Kcals:** 274 **Fat:** 15.5g **Saturated fat:** 5.5g **Carbs:** 14g **Sugar:** 8.3g **Fibre:** 5.1g **Protein:** 16.7g **Salt:** 0.9g **Allergens:** Eggs, milk

INGREDIENTS

6 eggs
200ml lactose-free milk
salt and freshly ground black pepper
160g/1 yellow pepper, diced
80g baby spinach, chopped
60g goats' cheese (or your preferred cheese)
1 tbsp rapeseed oil, plus extra for greasing
340g/2 large parsnips, peeled and thinly sliced lengthways

WHAT TO DO

1 Preheat the oven to 165°C. Lightly grease two silicone muffin trays.
2 Whisk together the eggs, milk and some salt and pepper in a bowl until combined. Add the yellow pepper, spinach and cheese and mix well, then spoon into the greased muffin trays. Bake in the oven for 15–20 minutes, until golden on top.
3 Meanwhile, heat the oil in a frying pan set over a high heat. Fry the parsnip strips in batches on both sides for 1–2 minutes, until golden brown. Season with freshly ground black pepper.
4 Remove the mini frittatas from the trays and serve with the parsnip chips.

Preparation time: 10 minutes
Cooking time: 20 minutes
Serves: 6–8

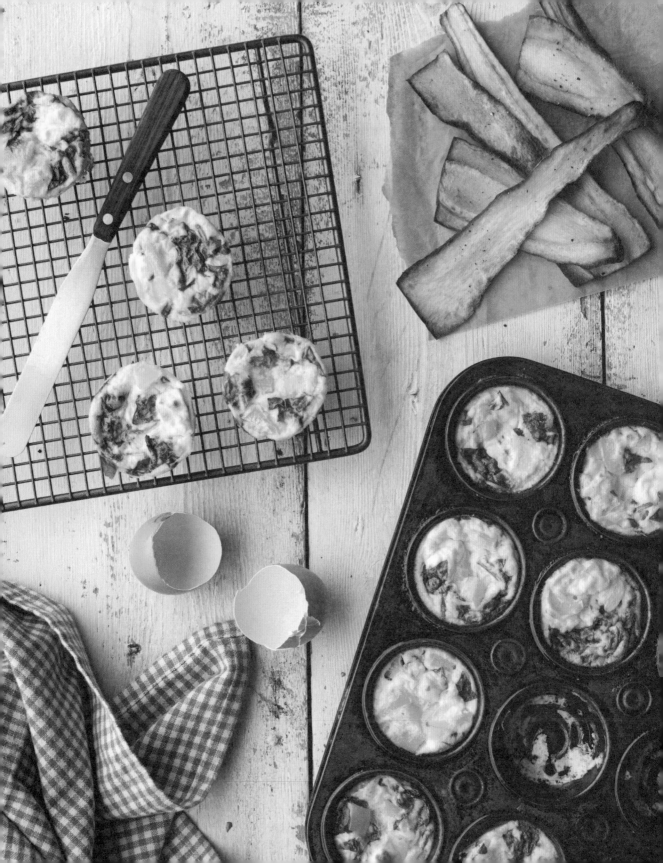

Chunky Chilli con Quorn

This dish has all the taste of a classic chilli, but with fewer calories and less saturated fat.
It's also a good source of protein for vegetarians.

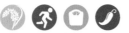

Portion size: 416g **Kcals:** 419 **Fat:** 5.8g **Saturated fat:** 0.9g **Carbs:** 66g **Sugar:** 13.4g
Fibre: 11.8g **Protein:** 18.5g **Salt:** 1.1g **Allergens:** Eggs, milk, may contain soya

INGREDIENTS

1 tbsp garlic-infused oil
260g/4 medium carrots, cut into
    chunks
320g/1 courgette, cut into chunks
300g Quorn mince
2 tsp ground cumin
1 tsp chilli powder (optional)
1 tsp smoked paprika
1 tsp dried basil
½ tsp ground cinnamon
1 x 400g tin of chopped tomatoes
2 tbsp tomato purée
260g brown rice

WHAT TO DO

1 Heat the oil in a pan set over a medium heat. Add the carrots
   and courgette and cook for 4–5 minutes, until soft. Add the
   Quorn mince along with all the dried herbs and spices and
   continue to cook for 2–3 minutes, until the Quorn is starting to
   turn brown.
2 Add the tinned tomatoes and tomato purée. Bring to the boil,
   then reduce the heat and simmer for 20 minutes.
3 Meanwhile, cook the rice as per the packet instructions.
4 When cooked, remove the chilli from the heat and allow it to
   stand for 10 minutes to let the flavours blend. Serve with the
   rice.

Preparation time: 20 minutes
Cooking time: 30 minutes
Serves: 4

Nutty Feta Baked Potato

Eating the potato skins will maximise the fibre content of your meal, but only if you can tolerate them. To save time, the potatoes can be cooked in the microwave for 10–15 minutes (without the foil!). A gourmet baked potato!

Portion size: 352g **Kcals:** 419 **Fat:** 15.3g **Saturated fat:** 5.2g **Carbs:** 53g **Sugar:** 4.3g **Fibre:** 7.3g
Protein: 13.4g **Salt:** 0.8g **Allergens:** Tree nuts, milk

WHAT TO DO

1 Preheat the oven to 200°C.
2 Scrub the potatoes and cut an X into the top with a sharp knife. Wrap each potato separately in tin foil and bake in the oven for 1 hour.
3 Ten minutes from the end of the cooking time, spread the pine nuts on a baking sheet and toast in the oven, stirring occasionally, for 5–10 minutes, until golden brown.
4 Heat the olive oil in a large pan set over a high heat, then add the lemon zest and juice. Add the spinach and cook for 2–3 minutes, until wilted. Add the feta and stir until it begins to melt, then stir in the toasted pine nuts and the fresh herbs. Season with freshly ground black pepper.
5 To serve, unwrap the baked potatoes and push them open. Place one-quarter of the spinach mixture into each baked potato and season with another pinch of black pepper.

INGREDIENTS

1kg/approx. 4 baking potatoes
30g pine nuts
1 tbsp extra virgin olive oil
zest and juice of 1 lemon
200g spinach, chopped
120g feta, crumbled
1 tbsp chopped fresh mint or dill
freshly ground black pepper

Preparation time: 10 minutes
Cooking time: 15–60 minutes
Serves: 4

Stocks, Dressings, Dips, Spreads, Sides & Sauces

One of the toughest *challenges* of the low FODMAP diet is avoiding the ubiquitous supermarket sauces, jars and condiments. The *fail-safe* solutions in this chapter will tide you through the restrictive Stage 1 phase. The sun-dried *tomato pesto* and black olive tapenade are so tasty, quick and simple that they may even remain *firm favourites* in your recipe repertoire even after you've finished Stage 1.

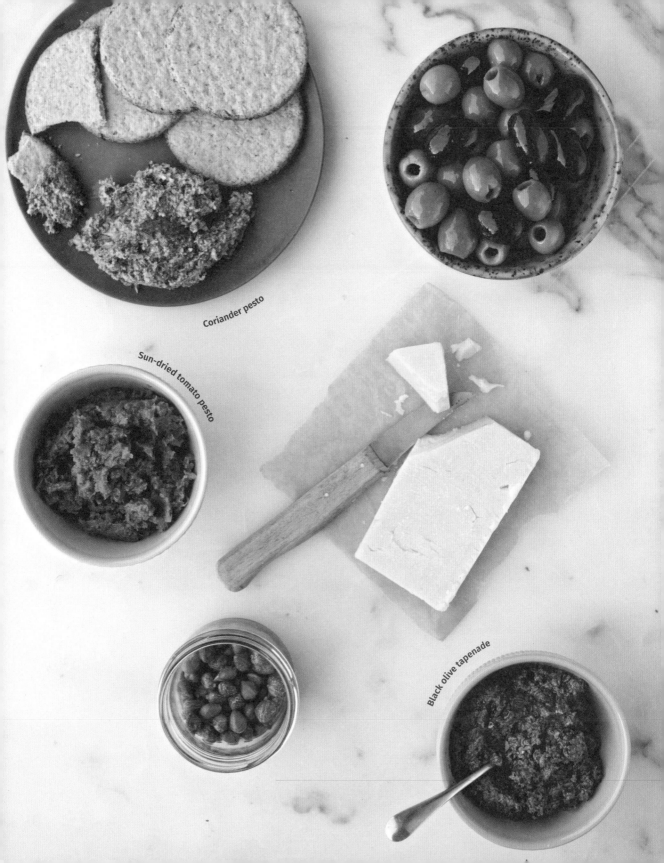

Coriander pesto

Sun-dried tomato pesto

Black olive tapenade

STOCK

Easy Chicken Stock

Most shop-bought stock or stock cubes contain onion and garlic alongside other FODMAPs such as gluten, lactose, yeast or flavour enhancers. Making up a large batch every now and then and freezing it in ready-to-go portions is recommended. If you make it while cooking another meal, it doesn't seem too laborious. **Making your own stock ensures you comply with low FODMAP advice as well as adding extra flavour to your meals.**

Portion size: 100ml **Kcals:** 16.3 **Fat:** 0.8g **Saturated fat:** 0.2g **Carbs:** 0g **Sugar:** 0g **Fibre:** 0g **Protein:** 2.3g
Salt: 0.4g **Allergens:** Celery

INGREDIENTS

1 tsp garlic-infused oil
1 x 2kg chicken carcass, cut up into 6–8 pieces, or leftover cooked chicken
240g/1 turnip, cut into chunks
180g/3 celery stalks, cut into chunks
130g/2 carrots, cut into chunks
handful of fresh herbs (parsley, thyme and rosemary work well)
handful of fresh chives, finely chopped
3 bay leaves
1 tsp whole black peppercorns
3 litres cold water
salt

WHAT TO DO

1 Heat the oil in a large stockpot. Place all the ingredients in the pot, cover with the cold water and season with salt. Bring to the boil, then reduce the heat and simmer, covered, for 1½–2 hours. As it cooks, skim any impurities off the surface.

2 When the cooking time is up, strain the stock into a large bowl. Pull off any meat left on the chicken for another use, such as salads or sandwiches, and discard the rest of the solids.

3 You can use the stock as it is and store it in the fridge for up to three days or freeze for up to three months for future use. Another tip is to reduce the stock by half by vigorously boiling it, uncovered, then allow to cool, pour into ice cube trays and freeze. When frozen, put the cubes into a ziplock bag and label with the date. When you want to use one, just put it in a jug and add boiling water to dissolve the cube. *Voilà* – lots of homemade chicken stock!

Preparation time: 15 minutes
Cooking time: 2 hours
Makes: 2 litres

Alternative Stock Cubes

This popular recipe does a great job of imitating shop-bought bouillon and it really jazzes up meals. It can be kept in the freezer to use when needed.

Portion size: 6g/1 cube **Kcals:** 6 **Fat:** 0.4g **Saturated fat:** 0.1g **Carbs:** 0.3g **Sugar:** 0.2g **Fibre:** 0.3g
Protein: 0.1g **Salt:** 0.02g **Allergens:** Sulphites

WHAT TO DO

1 Place the carrot, sun-dried tomatoes, spring onions, green pepper and radishes in a food processor and blend until all the ingredients are finely chopped. Add the fresh herbs, pepper and salt, if using, and blend again until you have a smooth paste.
2 This can be used immediately by using 1 teaspoon of the paste per 600ml water. Put the remainder into ice cube trays and freeze, then store the individual cubes in a ziplock bag for up to three months.

INGREDIENTS

70g/1 medium carrot, chopped into
    chunky pieces
30g/5 sun-dried tomatoes
20g/4 spring onions (green part only)
80g/½ green pepper, roughly chopped
34g/2 radishes, halved
1 tbsp chopped fresh chives
handful of fresh coriander
handful of fresh parsley
1 tsp ground white pepper
1 tsp salt (optional)

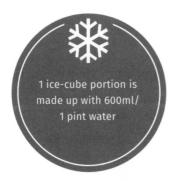

1 ice-cube portion is made up with 600ml/ 1 pint water

Preparation time: 15 minutes
Cooking time: N/A
Makes: 40 cubes

GRAVIES

Roasted Meat Gravy

There's nothing nicer than authentic gravy made from the juices of roasted meat. Combine it with stews, casseroles or to complement the ultimate Sunday roast.

Portion size: 100ml **Kcals:** 87 **Fat:** 0.2g **Saturated fat:** 0.02g **Carbs:** 21g **Sugar:** 0.01g **Fibre:** 0.5g **Protein:** 0.2g **Salt:** 1.9g **Allergens:** Celery

---

INGREDIENTS

3 tbsp water

1 tbsp cornflour

½ tsp gravy salt (a mixture of salt, cornflour and caramel)

200ml roast meat juices, strained

homemade low FODMAP stock (page 118), if necessary

WHAT TO DO

1 Place the cornflour and water in a saucepan set over a gentle heat and whisk together to make a paste. Stir in the gravy salt, then slowly stir in the strained meat juices, stirring continuously for about 10 minutes, until the gravy thickens. Add some FODMAP-friendly stock if the gravy is too thick.

2 Pour the gravy into a gravy boat and serve warm.

Preparation time: 2 minutes
Cooking time: 10 minutes
Serves: 2–4

Miso Gravy

This is different, but it works! Make sure you use a low FODMAP stock, such as the easy homemade chicken stock on page 118. If you don't want to use meat juices, use extra stock instead. This miso gravy goes well with chicken and potatoes. **Make sure to check that your miso paste has no garlic or onion added by checking the ingredients list of the product you buy.**

Portion size: 190ml **Kcals:** 47 **Fat:** 1.5g **Saturated fat:** 0.7g **Carbs:** 7.3g **Sugar:** 0.4g **Fibre:** 0.4g **Protein:** 0.6g **Salt:** 0.5g
Allergens: Soya, milk, may contain fish, may contain sulphites, may contain mustard, may contain celery

WHAT TO DO

1 Remove the meat from the roasting tray. Let the juices settle, then skim off the fat. You're aiming to get about 200ml.
2 Melt the butter in a heavy-based saucepan set over a medium heat. Add the cornflour and stir continuously until it has browned slightly.
3 Gradually add the miso paste, meat juices and stock. Keep stirring to ensure no bits stick to the bottom of the pan. Simmer for about 10 minutes, until the gravy thickens. Add more stock or water if it's too thick. Stir in the mustard, if using, and season before serving.

INGREDIENTS

200ml roasted meat juices, skimmed of all fat
1 tsp butter
1 tbsp cornflour
1 tbsp (1 sachet) miso paste
500ml homemade low FODMAP stock (page 118) (or the bullion on page 119 if you're in a hurry!)
½ tsp Dijon mustard (optional)
salt and freshly ground black pepper

Preparation time: 15 minutes
Cooking time: 15 minutes
Serves: 4

DRESSINGS

Salad Dressing

Homemade salad dressing is in every foodie's fridge. This dressing is richly flavoured from the zingy lemon/lime and refreshing mint leaves. One of the best things about making your own dressing is that you can tailor it according to your likes and dislikes. For more adventurous flavours, add some Tabasco sauce, mustard, chilli flakes, feta or blue cheese.

Portion size: 30ml **Kcals:** 18 **Fat:** 9g **Saturated fat:** 2.6g **Carbs:** 1.4g **Sugar:** 0.9g **Fibre:** 0.2g **Protein:** 0.1g
Salt: 0.5g **Allergens:** Sulphites

INGREDIENTS

6 tbsp olive oil
2 tbsp balsamic, red wine or white
   wine vinegar
1 tbsp lemon or lime juice
2.5cm piece of fresh ginger, peeled and
   chopped, or a handful of chopped
   fresh herbs, such as mint, parsley or
   coriander
salt and freshly ground black pepper

WHAT TO DO

1 Whisk all the ingredients together. Store in an airtight jar in the fridge for two or three days.

Preparation time: 5 minutes
Cooking time: N/A
Serves: 4

Chilli Lime Dressing

You don't have to spend ages preparing your salad jars for lunch at the office. The whole idea is to have your dressing made in minutes. Then all you have to do is turf in some roughly chopped salad vegetables and bite-sized pieces of protein. This simple spicy chilli dressing will give a kick to your greens and add buckets of flavour.

 Portion size: 30ml **Kcals:** 120 **Fat :**12.8g **Saturated fat:** 1.8g **Carbs:** 0.8g **Sugar:** 0.5g **Fibre:** 0.5g **Protein:** 0.4g
Salt: 1g **Allergens:** None

WHAT TO DO

1 Whisk all the ingredients together. Store in an airtight jar in the fridge for two or three days.

INGREDIENTS

2 tbsp extra virgin olive oil
2 tbsp fresh lime juice
1 tsp ground cumin
pinch of chilli flakes
salt and freshly ground black pepper

Preparation time: 2 minutes
Cooking time: N/A
Serves: 2

Sesame Lemon Dressing

This sesame Asian dressing is so delicious and yummy it will liven up your salad leaves no end. In fact, everyone who gets a whiff of it as you shake it up and empty your salad jar will want some, so beware!

 Portion size: 30ml **Kcals:** 81 **Fat:** 5.3g **Saturated fat:** 0.8g **Carbs:** 4.2g **Sugar:** 3g **Fibre:** 1.3g **Protein:** 1.3g **Salt:** 1.4g
Allergens: Sesame, sulphites

INGREDIENTS

1 tbsp rice wine vinegar
1 tbsp lemon juice
1 tbsp tahini
1 tsp sesame oil
¼ tsp dried oregano
pinch of chilli flakes
salt and freshly ground black pepper

WHAT TO DO

1 Whisk all the ingredients together. Store in an airtight jar in the fridge for two or three days.

Preparation time: 3 minutes
Cooking time: N/A
Serves: 1

Black Olive Tapenade

Why buy tapenade when this is so easy to make? This also works well with green olives.

Portion size: 26g **Kcals:** 74 **Fat:** 7.7g **Saturated fat:** 1.1g **Carbs:** 0.1g **Sugar:** 0.1g **Fibre:** 0.7g **Protein:** 0.5g **Salt:** 0.8g
Allergens: Mustard, fish

WHAT TO DO

1 Place the olives, anchovies (if using) and capers in a food processor and blend until finely chopped.
2 With the blender on a low speed, slowly add the oil in a steady stream until well combined and a smooth paste has formed.
3 Finally, add the parsley and Dijon mustard and blend for a few seconds, until combined.
4 Transfer to an airtight container and pour over a thin layer of oil to cover the tapenade surface to keep it fresh. This will keep in the fridge for up to four days.

INGREDIENTS

175g pitted black olives
3–4 tinned anchovy fillets, drained (optional)
1 tbsp drained capers
4 tbsp garlic-infused extra virgin olive oil
handful of fresh parsley
½ tsp Dijon mustard

Preparation time: 10 minutes
Cooking time: N/A
Makes: 1 jar

Baba Ghanoush

This beautiful Middle Eastern-inspired aubergine dip is best served with gluten-free pitta bread, oat crackers or vegetable crudités.

 Portion size: 53g **Kcals:** 66 **Fat:** 6.1g **Saturated fat:** 0.9g **Carbs:** 1g **Sugar:** 0.9g **Fibre:** 1.1g **Protein:** 1g
Salt: 0g **Allergens:** Sesame

INGREDIENTS

250g/1 small aubergine
juice of ½ lemon
2 tbsp garlic-infused olive oil, plus
    extra for rubbing and drizzling
1 tbsp tahini
1 tbsp chopped fresh mint
freshly ground black pepper

WHAT TO DO

1 Preheat the oven to 220°C.
2 Prick the aubergine all over with a fork. Rub with a little oil and place on a baking tray. Roast in the oven for about 20 minutes, turning halfway through, until the skin is blackened and the flesh feels soft when you press it. Remove from the oven and allow to cool – the longer the skin stays on, the smokier it will taste.
3 Slice the cooled aubergine in half lengthways. Scoop out the flesh into a bowl and discard the skins. If it appears very moist, place in a sieve and squeeze out as much liquid from the flesh as you can.
4 In a separate large bowl, mix together the lemon juice, oil, tahini, most of the mint and some black pepper.
5 Mash the aubergine and add it to the other ingredients in the large bowl. Or if it's easier, you can blend everything in a blender or food processor for a few seconds until all the ingredients are combined.
6 Place in a serving dish. Finish with a drizzle of olive oil and garnish with the remaining mint leaves.

Preparation time: 10 minutes
Cooking time: 20 minutes
Serves: 6 (makes 1 bowl)

Sun-Dried Tomato Pesto

Perfect for making lazy-person pasta after work or as a pizza sauce. **When buying jars of sun-dried tomatoes in oil, make sure there is no onion or garlic on the ingredients list.**

Portion size: 27g **Kcals:** 129 **Fat:** 13.3g **Saturated fat:** 1.8g
Carbs: 0.7g **Sugar:** 0.4g **Fibre:** 1.8g **Protein:** 0.5g **Salt:** 0.7g
Allergens: Sulphites

INGREDIENTS

54g/1 jar of sun-dried tomatoes in oil,
    drained
2 tbsp capers
1 tbsp white wine vinegar
2 tbsp garlic-infused olive oil
freshly ground black pepper

WHAT TO DO

1 Put the sun-dried tomatoes, capers and vinegar in a food processor and blend. Slowly pour the oil in until it reaches a consistency you like. You may need to scrape down the sides of the bowl once or twice.
2 Season to taste with freshly ground black pepper before serving.

Coriander Pesto

This delicious and flavoursome alternative to basil pesto goes really well with fish, chicken, pasta or on 100% sourdough spelt toast.

Portion size: 42g **Kcals:** 193 **Fat:** 20g **Saturated fat:** 2.2g
Carbs: 1.2g **Sugar:** 0.8g **Fibre:** 1.4g **Protein:** 1.6g **Salt:** 0.01g
Allergens: Tree nuts

INGREDIENTS

60g pecans
large handful of fresh coriander
juice of 1 lime
2½ tbsp garlic-infused olive oil
freshly ground black pepper

WHAT TO DO

1 Put the pecans, coriander, lime juice and half of the oil in a food processor and blend until smooth. Slowly pour in the remaining oil until it reaches a consistency you like. You may need to scrape down the sides of the bowl once or twice.
2 Season to taste with freshly ground black pepper before serving.

Preparation time: 10 minutes
Cooking time: N/A
Serves: 4

Preparation time: 10 minutes
Cooking time: N/A
Serves: 4

SIDES
Low FODMAP Coleslaw

This expected addition to a BBQ or buffet is really easy to make. It also goes well with a strong cheese like Camembert or blue cheese. **Although cabbage gets a bad name for those who suffer with IBS, red and white cabbage are actually on the allowed FODMAP list, as they are deemed to be low FODMAP. Savoy cabbage is the one to restrict to <35g while following Stage 1.**

 Portion size: 128g **Kcals:** 56 **Fat:** 0.6g **Saturated fat:** 0.1g **Carbs:** 6.6g **Sugar:** 5.9g **Fibre:** 2.9g **Protein:** 4.5g
Salt: 0.1g **Allergens:** Mustard, milk, sulphites

INGREDIENTS
200g low-fat Greek yogurt
2 tbsp white wine or rice vinegar
2 tsp Dijon mustard
1 tsp caster sugar
200g/½ small red cabbage, core
    removed and thinly shredded
200g/½ small white cabbage, core
    removed and thinly shredded
120g/1 large carrot, shredded
1 large handful of fresh parsley leaves,
    chopped
1 tsp poppy seeds
salt and freshly ground black pepper

WHAT TO DO
1 Place the Greek yogurt, vinegar, mustard and sugar in a small bowl and mix well.
2 Place the shredded cabbages and carrot in a large serving bowl and pour the dressing over the top. Add the parsley and poppy seeds and toss to thoroughly combine. Season to taste and chill before serving.

Preparation time: 10 minutes
Cooking time: N/A
Serves: 6

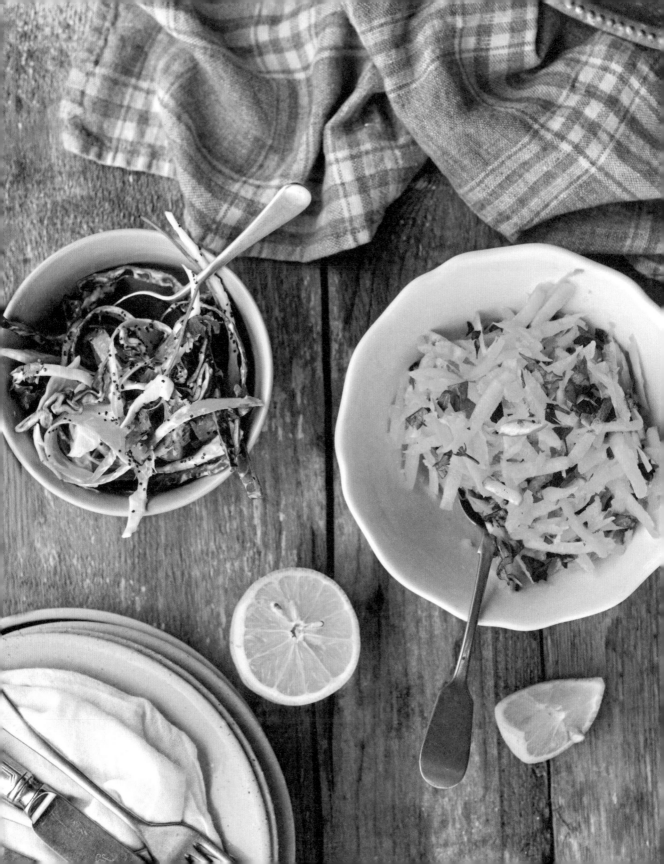

Carrot Slaw

For those who want a deliciously crunchy coleslaw alternative or who don't 'do' cabbage!

Portion size: 82g **Kcals:** 109 **Fat:** 9.2g
Saturated fat: 1.4g **Carbs:** 4.8g
Sugar: 4.4g **Fibre:** 2.5g **Protein:** 0.4g
Salt: 0.05g **Allergens:** None

INGREDIENTS

3 tbsp extra virgin olive oil
1 tbsp freshly squeezed lemon juice
240g/2 large carrots, grated
34g/2 radishes, grated (optional)
2 tbsp chopped fresh parsley
freshly ground black pepper

WHAT TO DO

1 Whisk together the oil and lemon juice.
2 Place the carrots and radishes (if using) in a serving bowl. Pour over the dressing and toss to combine. Add the parsley and toss again.
3 Season to taste with freshly ground black pepper before serving.

Preparation time: 10 minutes
Cooking time: N/A
Serves: 4

Carrot and Orange Salad

A delightfully refreshing winter salad that goes great with cold turkey or ham – perfect for using up after Christmas dinner!

Portion size: 144g **Kcals:** 133 **Fat:** 8.1g
Saturated fat: 1.3g **Carbs:** 10.5g **Sugar:** 9.6g
Fibre: 5g **Protein:** 1.7g **Salt:** 0.5g
Allergens: Sesame

INGREDIENTS

2 tbsp sesame seeds
2 tbsp extra virgin olive oil
2 tbsp orange juice
1 tbsp lemon juice
½ tbsp ground cumin
½ tbsp ground cinnamon
salt and freshly ground black pepper
450g carrots, coarsely grated
240g/4 satsumas, peeled and cut crossways into slices, then into small segments
handful of fresh coriander, parsley and/or mint leaves, roughly chopped

WHAT TO DO

1 Preheat the oven to 180°C.
2 Scatter the sesame seeds on a baking tray and toast in the oven for about 5 minutes.
3 Whisk together the olive oil, orange juice, lemon juice, cumin, cinnamon and a pinch of salt and pepper in a large bowl. Add the grated carrots, satsuma segments and herbs and lightly toss.
4 Sprinkle the toasted sesame seeds over the top and mix through just before serving.

Preparation time: 15 minutes
Cooking time: 5 minutes
Serves: 5

Julienned Carrot, Cucumber and Herb Salad

This crisp, fresh side salad goes with just about everything! Julienne is a technique of cutting your vegetables into long, thin strips, like matchsticks, and gives your salad a new standout look. Use a spiraliser or a vegetable peeler to create long, thin ribbons if you don't have time to julienne your vegetables.

  Portion size: 160g **Kcals:** 71 **Fat:** 0.7g **Saturated fat:** 0.1g **Carbs:** 12.5g **Sugar:** 11g **Fibre:** 2.6g **Protein:** 1.2g **Salt:** 0.2g **Allergens:** Sulphites

WHAT TO DO

1 To make the dressing, heat the vinegar and maple syrup in a small non-reactive saucepan. Add the chilli and stir until the syrup has dissolved, then remove from the heat and allow to cool.
2 In a large bowl, toss the julienned or spiralised vegetables through the dressing along with the coriander leaves and refrigerate.
3 Just before serving, the mint leaves can be chiffonaded or neatly chopped before you stir them through the salad.

INGREDIENTS

200g/3 medium carrots, julienned, spiralised or peeled into ribbons
300g/1 cucumber, deseeded and julienned, spiralised or peeled into ribbons
handful of fresh coriander leaves
handful of fresh mint leaves

For the dressing:
60ml rice vinegar
1 tbsp maple syrup
½ red chilli, deseeded and finely chopped

Preparation time: 10 minutes
Cooking time: 5 minutes
Serves: 4

Fennel, Orange, Feta and Pomegranate Salad with Rocket

Feta, Cheddar, mozzarella, Brie, Camembert, blue, Edam and goats' cheese are all low in lactose and can be included in a low FODMAP plan. This protein-rich cheese salad is delicious served with a simple piece of 100% sourdough spelt bread. **Fennel adds a depth of flavour, but less than 3 tablespoons is recommended per sitting, as more can cause symptoms.**

Portion size: 217g **Kcals:** 243 **Fat:** 17g **Saturated fat:** 7.8g **Carbs:** 11g **Sugar:** 10.8g **Fibre:** 3.6g **Protein:** 9.6g
Salt: 1.3g **Allergens:** Milk

INGREDIENTS

160g/1 medium orange
80g/1 small bulb of fennel, trimmed
50g/½ small pomegranate (less than ½ small pomegranate recommended)
1 tbsp extra virgin olive oil
1 tsp lemon juice
salt and freshly ground black pepper
100g feta, crumbled into small pieces
25g rocket

WHAT TO DO

1 Peel the orange and separate each segment, then cut into pieces and place in a bowl. Squeeze the orange segment casings over the bowl to release any extra juice.
2 Cut the fennel in half lengthways and finely slice into paper-thin lengths, then mix into the orange segments.
3 Hold the pomegranate half over the bowl so you don't lose any juices and pull out the pink seeds with a teaspoon, discarding the cream-coloured membrane. Mix in the olive oil and lemon juice and season to taste.
4 When ready to serve, mix in the crumbled feta and rocket and divide the salad between two plates.

Preparation time: 15 minutes
Cooking time: N/A
Serves: 2

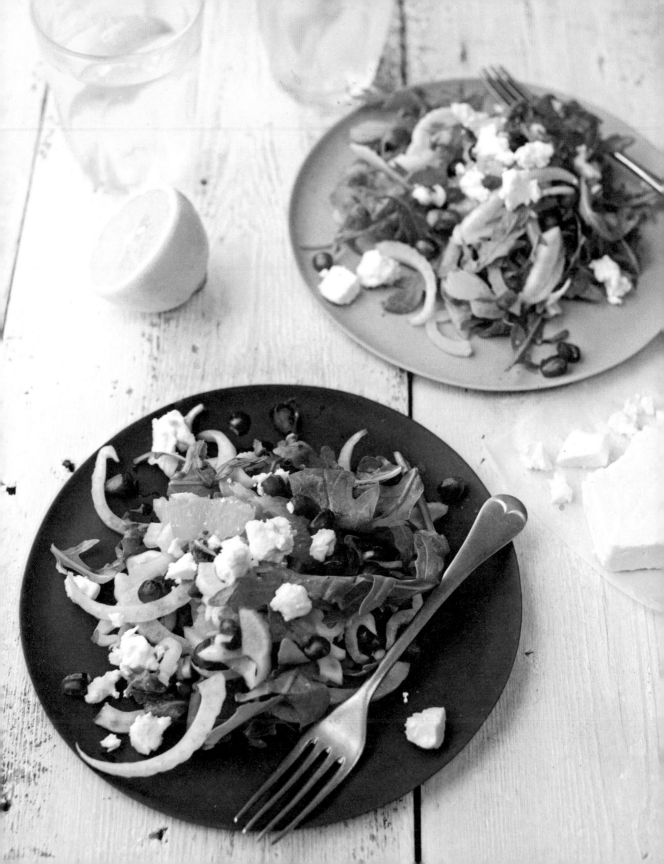

SAUCES

Sweet Chilli Dipping Sauce

This savoury dipping sauce can be used in many recipes, such as fish cakes and homemade chicken nuggets, and can even be used on pizza instead of tomato sauce.

 Portion size: 74g **Kcals:** 80 **Fat:** 0.1g
Saturated fat: 0g **Carbs:** 20g **Sugar:** 19.3g
Fibre: 0.2g **Protein:** 0.3g **Salt:** 0.3g
Allergens: None

INGREDIENTS

2 tbsp light brown sugar
4 tbsp rice vinegar
2 tbsp water
pinch of salt
½ red chilli, deseeded and finely chopped, plus extra
   to garnish
chopped fresh coriander, to garnish

WHAT TO DO

1 Place a small saucepan (not stainless steel – vinegar reacts with it and will give the sauce a metallic taste) over a medium heat. Add the vinegar, water and brown sugar and stir until the sugar has dissolved. Let it thicken up a little over a gentle heat. Add the finely chopped chilli and salt to taste.
2 Serve the dip in a ramekin and garnish with some fresh coriander and extra chilli.

Preparation time: 2 minutes
Cooking time: 10–15 minutes
Serves: 2

Red Curry Paste

Soy, oyster and fish sauces are suitable when following a low FODMAP diet. Minor wheat ingredients in these sauces aren't a problem. Use these sauces along with coriander, ginger, suitable vegetables and rice for a healthy, low FODMAP, Asian-inspired meal.

 Portion size: 10g **Kcals:** 19 **Fat:** 1.8g
Saturated fat: 0.3g **Carbs:** 0.3g **Sugar:** 0.3g
Fibre: 0.2g **Protein:** 0.2g **Salt:** 0.2g
Allergens: Fish

INGREDIENTS

40g/8 spring onions (green part only), chopped
4 dried red chillies
juice of 1 lime
1 tbsp peeled, chopped fresh ginger
4 tsp garlic-infused oil
4 tsp Thai fish sauce
2 tsp chopped fresh coriander
1 tsp lemon juice
1 tsp coriander seeds
½ tsp cumin seeds
½ tsp ground white pepper

WHAT TO DO

1 Place all the ingredients in a food processor and blitz to a smooth consistency. Keep the curry paste in an airtight container for a couple of weeks in your fridge or for a couple of months in your freezer.

Preparation time: 10 minutes
Cooking time: N/A
Makes: 280g/10 dessertspoons

Tomato and Basil Pasta Sauce

Tomato sauce is the foundation of so many good dishes, such as Bolognese, lasagna or stews, or it can be simply spooned over cooked gluten-free pasta with plenty of freshly grated Parmesan cheese. **Balsamic vinegar is used in the recipe but only in small amounts. The FODMAP cut-off is a maximum of 1 tablespoon per sitting. Remember, most shop-bought tomato sauces contain high FODMAP ingredients.** You can make this in large batches and freeze to use when needed.

Portion size: 114g **Kcals:** 87 **Fat:** 6.4g **Saturated fat:** 0.9g **Carbs:** 5.5g **Sugar:** 5.3g **Fibre:** 1g **Protein:** 1.3g **Salt:** 0.02g
Allergens: May contain sulphites

WHAT TO DO

1 Heat the oil in a saucepan set over a low heat. Add the spring onions and gently cook for 1–2 minutes.
2 Stir in the tomatoes, balsamic vinegar, sugar and chilli flakes (if using). Bring to a simmer and cook slowly for 1 hour.
3 Stir in the basil and season to taste with salt and pepper. This sauce can be left chunky or blended in a food processor for a smooth sauce.

INGREDIENTS

2 tbsp garlic-infused extra virgin olive oil
10g/2 spring onions (green part only)
1 x 400g tin of chopped tomatoes or passata
2 tsp balsamic vinegar
1 tsp caster sugar
½ tsp dried chilli flakes (optional)
1 large handful of basil leaves, torn into small pieces
salt and freshly ground black pepper

Preparation time: 10 minutes
Cooking time: 1 hour
Serves: 4

Chilli Oil

This combination of chillies, coriander and garlic-infused oil makes this a perfect oil to give any dish an extra kick.

   Portion size: 10g **Kcals:** 46 **Fat:** 5g **Saturated fat:** 0.7g **Carbs:** 0.2g **Sugar:** 0.2g **Fibre:** 0.1g
Protein: 0.1g **Salt:** 0.0g **Allergens:** None

INGREDIENTS

2–3 fresh red chillies, deseeded
    and halved
160g/1 red pepper, chopped
handful of fresh coriander
250ml garlic-infused oil

WHAT TO DO

1 Place all the ingredients in a food processor and blend together. Store in an airtight container in the fridge for up to one week.

Preparation time: 2 minutes
Cooking time: N/A
Makes: 250ml

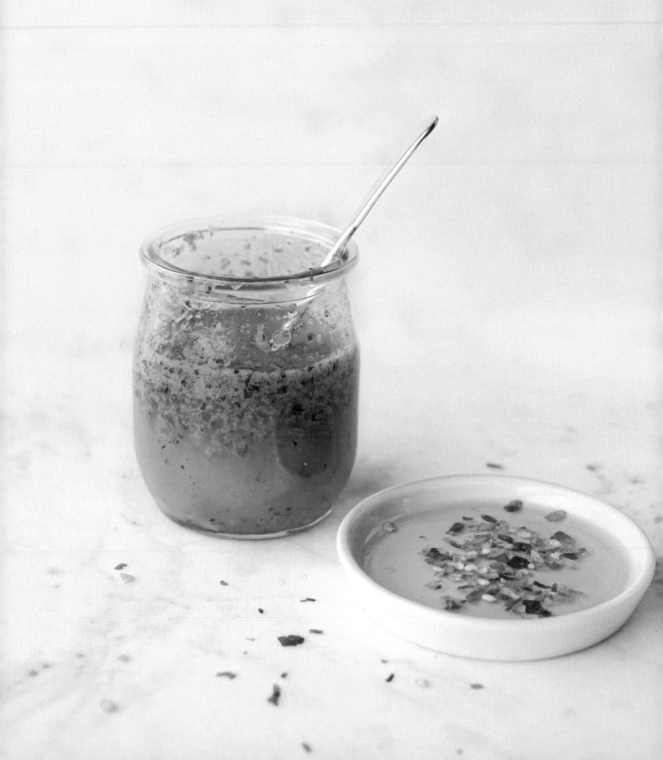

Dessert

A *treat* chapter because we are all human! Great for parties, birthdays and any other *special* occasions, some are even low in calories if you fancy a nibble of something *sweet*.

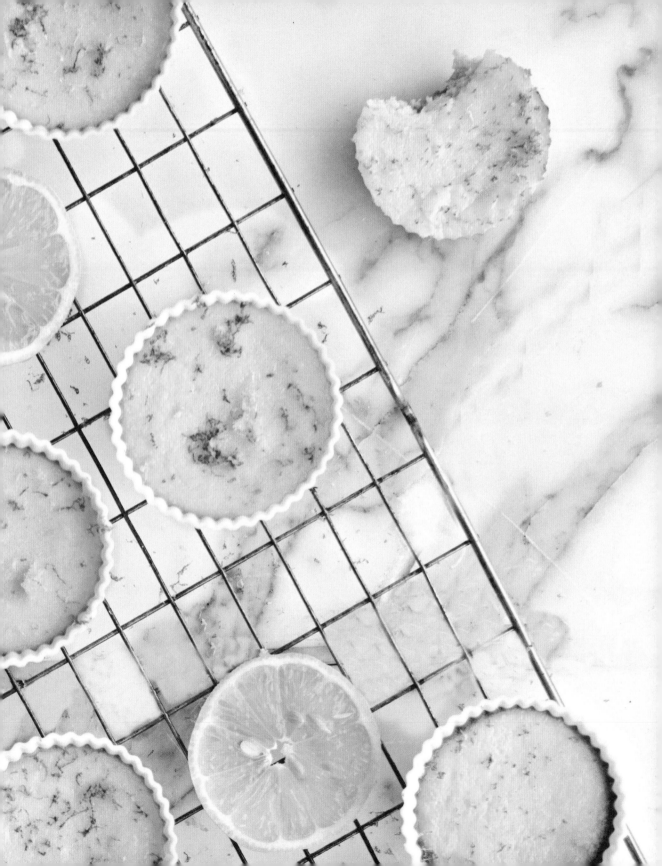

Baked Camembert with Poppy Seed Breadsticks

Use a whole wheat bread mix to increase the fibre intake of this dessert/snack.

Portion size: 95g **Kcals:** 297 **Fat:** 19g **Saturated fat:** 7.4g **Carbs:** 19.2g **Sugar:** 0.5g **Fibre:** 1.7g **Protein:** 11.5g **Salt:** 0.7g
Allergens: Milk, may contain soya, may contain lupin

INGREDIENTS

250g Camembert
2 sprigs of fresh rosemary

For the breadsticks:
130g gluten-free bread mix
½ tsp xanthan gum
2 tbsp poppy seeds
75ml water
3 tbsp olive oil
1 egg, beaten

WHAT TO DO

1 Preheat the oven to 200°C.
2 Place the cheese, still in its box but with the lid off, on a baking tray. Pierce the top of the cheese a few times and stick the rosemary sprigs into the slits. Bake in the oven for 20 minutes.
3 Meanwhile, to make the breadsticks, put the flour, xanthan gum and 1 tablespoon of the poppy seeds in a food processor and blend for about 10 seconds to combine. Add the water and oil and blend until the mixture comes together.
4 Lightly dust your work surface with a little gluten-free flour and lightly oil a baking tray. Tip the dough out onto the floured surface and knead into a ball. Roll into a rectangle, then cut into 2.5cm-wide strips. Twist each strip gently and arrange on the oiled baking tray. Sprinkle with the rest of the poppy seeds.
5 Brush each stick with the beaten egg before placing in the oven and baking for about 10–15 minutes, until browned, or up 20 minutes for a crispier breadstick. Allow to cool on a wire rack.
6 Serve the breadsticks with the warm, gooey cheese.

Preparation time: 15 minutes
Cooking time: 20 minutes
Serves: 6

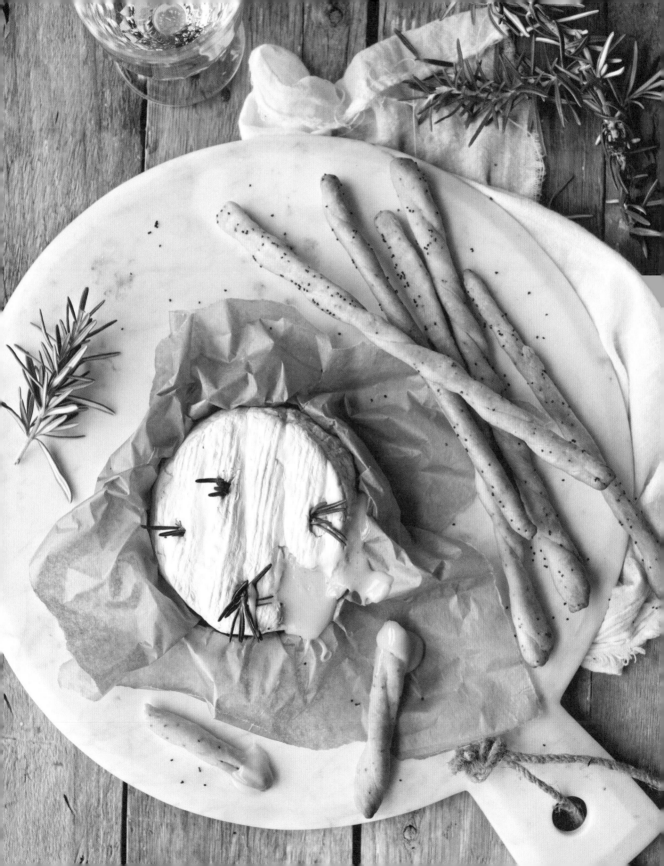

Gooey Chocolate Beetroot Brownies

These little gems are dark, rich and ideal for a FODMAPer's birthday. **Keep to one portion so that you stay within the guidelines for beetroot (<20g per serving).** Remember, the smaller the slice, the lower the calorie content!

Portion size: 70g **Kcals:** 273 **Fat:** 17.6g **Saturated fat:** 10.6g **Carbs:** 24g **Sugar:** 19.7g **Fibre:** 2.1g **Protein:** 3.3g
Salt: 0.4g **Allergens:** Eggs, may contain milk, may contain soya, may contain gluten, may contain nuts

INGREDIENTS

300g peeled, pre-cooked beetroots
250g dark chocolate, broken
    into pieces
250g butter, softened
300g caster sugar
3 medium eggs
75g gluten-free plain flour
50g cocoa powder
½ tsp xanthan powder
½ tsp baking powder
pinch of salt

WHAT TO DO

1 Preheat the oven to 180°C. Line a 33cm x 25cm baking pan or dish with non-stick baking paper.
2 Place the pre-cooked beetroot in a food processor and blend for a few minutes, until a smooth purée forms. Set to one side.
3 Melt the chocolate in a heatproof bowl set over a saucepan of simmering water or in the microwave and set aside.
4 Cream the butter in a food mixer until soft. Add the sugar and continue to mix until it turns light and fluffy.
5 Beat the eggs gently in a separate small bowl, then gradually add to the creamed butter mixture, beating all the time.
6 Beat in the puréed beetroot and melted chocolate, then sift in the remaining ingredients and fold in until fully combined.
7 Pour the batter into the prepared baking tin and even out the top with a spatula. Bake in the oven for 30–35 minutes, until the centre is almost set but still wobbles when you gently shake the tin.
8 Remove from the oven and place on a wire rack to cool. Allow to cool completely in the tin before carefully removing the brownies and cutting into squares to serve.

Preparation time: 15 minutes
Cooking time: 45 minutes
Makes: 20

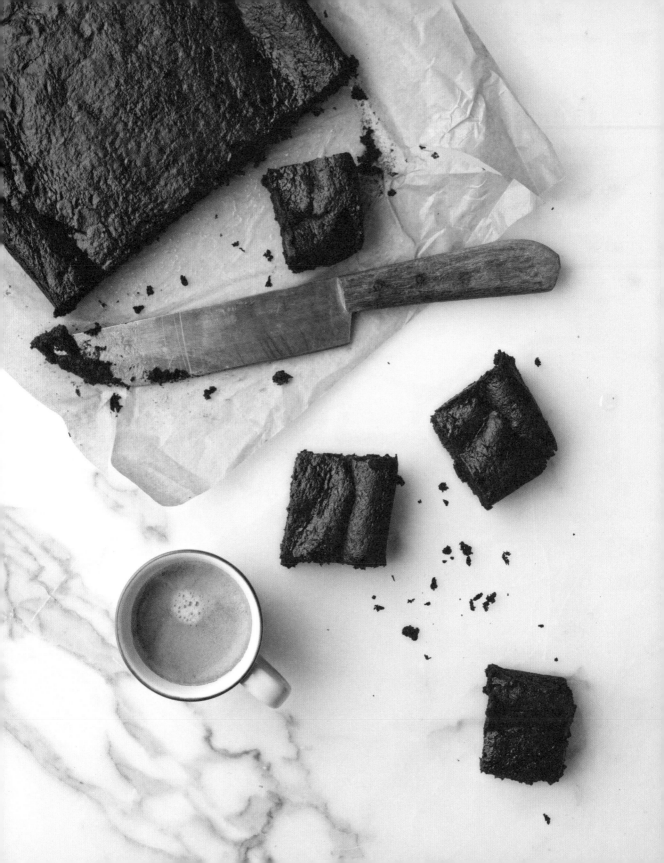

Chocolate Raspberry Pretend Mousse

A healthier take on a cream-based mousse, but still indulgent! **You can use most berries (exclude blackberries) or a berry mix in this recipe.**

Portion size: 133g **Kcals:** 214 **Fat:** 13.9g **Saturated fat:** 7.5g **Carbs:** 13.2g **Sugar:** 11.6g **Fibre:** 4.4g **Protein:** 5.9g
Salt: 0.2g **Allergens:** Soya, may contain milk, may contain nuts

INGREDIENTS

150g dark chocolate, broken
    into small pieces
500g plain or vanilla soya yogurt
2 tbsp maple syrup
1 tsp vanilla extract
100g fresh or frozen raspberries
    (thawed and drained if frozen)

WHAT TO DO

1 Place the chocolate pieces in a heatproof bowl set over a saucepan of simmering water, stirring often until it melts, or melt in the microwave, which takes about 1 minute. Allow to cool for about 10 minutes, then mix in the yogurt, maple syrup and vanilla. Fold in most of the raspberries.

2 Spoon the mousse into six ramekins and top with the remaining raspberries. Refrigerate for at least 30 minutes before serving.

Preparation time: 15 minutes
Cooking time: At least 30 minutes in the fridge
Serves: 6

Nutty Biscotti

These are delectable biscuits for a special occasion. **Be careful not to go over the 10 hazelnuts (15g) per portion in one sitting, though!**

Portion size: 28g **Kcals:** 110 **Fat:** 3.6g **Saturated fat:** 1.1g **Carbs:** 17.4g **Sugar:** 5.8g **Fibre:** 0.9g **Protein:** 1.6g **Salt:** 0.2g **Allergens:** Tree nuts, eggs, may contain soya, may contain lupin, may contain sulphites

WHAT TO DO

1 Preheat the oven to 200°C. Lightly grease a baking tray with oil and dust with a sprinkle of flour.
2 Separate the eggs into two bowls: one bowl with the egg whites, the other with the egg yolks.
3 Whisk the egg whites while gradually sifting in the icing sugar.
4 Lightly beat the egg yolks, then add them to the sugary egg whites, beating until the mixture is fluffy and stiff. Sift in the flour and baking powder and fold until combined. Stir in the chocolate, nuts and vanilla extract.
5 Use your hands to mould the dough into two or three logs and place on the prepared tray. Bake for 5 minutes, then reduce the heat to 160°C and bake for 15–20 minutes more, until the logs are lightly golden.
6 Remove from the oven and slice as thinly as possible without them crumbling. Place the biscuits back on the tray and return to the oven to bake for 5–10 minutes, until crispy. Cool on a wire rack. The biscuits will keep in an airtight container for two to three weeks.

INGREDIENTS

2 medium eggs
150g icing sugar
400g gluten-free white flour
2 tsp baking powder
80g dark chocolate, chopped into small pieces
40g hazelnuts, chopped into small pieces
40g macadamias
1 tsp vanilla extract

Preparation time: 15 minutes
Cooking time: 35–40 minutes
Makes: 30

Easy Rhubarb Crumble

Rest assured that if you make this, it will be devoured! **This is best served hot with cow's milk yogurt, soya yogurt or up to 50g of Greek or cow's milk yogurt.**

Portion size: 169g **Kcals:** 311 **Fat:** 13.4g **Saturated fat:** 7g **Carbs:** 43g **Sugar:** 30g **Fibre:** 4.6g **Protein:** 3.4g
Salt: 0.1g **Allergens:** Sesame, milk, may contain soya, may contain lupin, may contain gluten if oats are used

INGREDIENTS

150g light brown sugar

90g oats or gluten-free flour (or a
    combination of both)

2 tbsp mixed seeds

½ tsp ground nutmeg

75g butter, chilled and cut into small
    pieces

500g rhubarb

2 tbsp water

2 tbsp maple syrup

2 tsp ground cinnamon

125g frozen raspberries

WHAT TO DO

1 Preheat the oven to 180°C. Grease a 25cm x 18cm
baking dish.

2 In a medium bowl, mix the sugar, oats or flour, seeds and
nutmeg together. With your hands, work in the butter until
large, moist clumps form. Set aside.

3 Cut the rhubarb into 2.5–5cm pieces. Place in a saucepan
with the water, maple syrup and cinnamon and simmer for
about 10 minutes. Add the raspberries and stew gently for
another 10 minutes.

4 Spread the stewed rhubarb and raspberries into the
greased dish, then spoon the crumble topping over the
fruit. Bake in the oven for 25 minutes, until the crumble is
golden brown and the fruit is bubbling.

Preparation time: 15 minutes
Cooking time: 35–40 minutes
Serves: 6

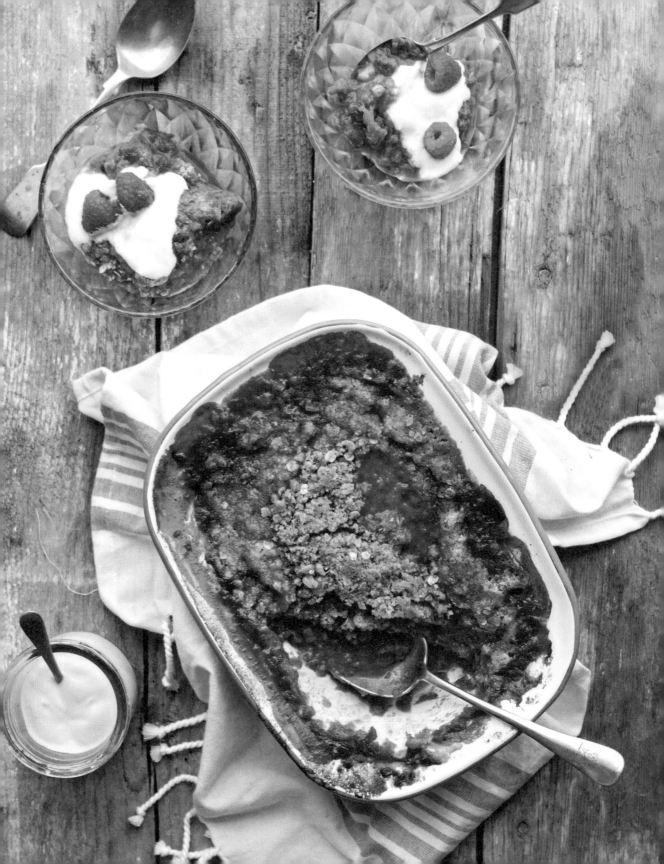

Beautiful Berry Mess

Everyone loves Eton mess, but this no-cook alternative is pretty good too! **Be careful to stick to the correct portion size of Greek yogurt, as outlined in the recipe (<50g per serving).**

  Portion size: 229g **Kcals:** 216 **Fat:** 4g **Saturated fat:** 2.3g **Carbs:** 30g **Sugar:** 29g **Fibre:** 6.1g **Protein:** 7.2g **Salt:** 0.1g **Allergens:** Milk, eggs, may contain gluten, may contain sulphites

INGREDIENTS

200g blueberries

200g strawberries

200g raspberries

1 tbsp maple syrup

200g Greek yogurt

2 tbsp Triple Sec or Grand Marnier
    (optional)

1 tsp grated lemon zest

1 tsp vanilla extract

52g/4 meringue nests, broken
    into pieces

WHAT TO DO

1 Combine the berries and maple syrup in a large bowl, keeping back a few whole berries for decoration. Mash the berries with the back of a spoon or fork until some juice seeps out.

2 In another bowl, mix the yogurt with the Triple Sec, if using, lemon zest and vanilla.

3 Add the meringue pieces and the berries to the yogurt mixture and gently fold until streaks of berry juice swirl through the yogurt.

4 Spoon into glass dishes and decorate with the reserved whole berries. Serve straight away or keep chilled in the fridge before serving.

Preparation time: 15 minutes
Cooking time: N/A
Serves: 4

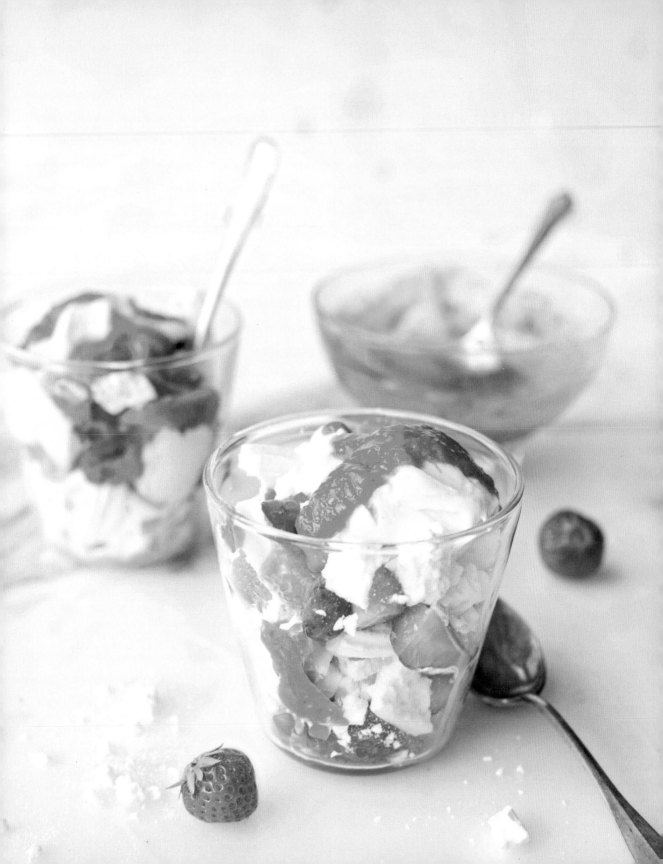

Banana and Pineapple Fritters

An old-school favourite! As bananas and pineapple are lovely and sweet, there is no need to add extra sugar in this dessert.

 Portion size: 162g **Kcals:** 227 **Fat:** 3.9g **Saturated fat:** 0.7g **Carbs:** 43g **Sugar:** 17.3g **Fibre:** 2.6g **Protein:** 3.3g
Salt: 0.2g **Allergens:** Milk, may contain soya, may contain lupin

INGREDIENTS

200g/2 medium bananas, cut in half lengthways
120g gluten-free flour
1 tsp ground cinnamon
150ml lactose-free milk
1 tbsp olive oil
160g/1 tin of pineapple chunks in natural juice, drained
1 tsp icing sugar, for dusting
1 scoop of dairy-free or soya ice cream, to serve

WHAT TO DO

1 Coat the bananas lightly with a little of the flour. Sift the remaining flour into a bowl with the cinnamon. Make a well in the centre and add the milk gradually. Mix to a smooth, thick consistency.

2 Heat the oil in a pan set over a high heat. Working in batches, dip the bananas and the pineapple chunks into the batter, shaking off any excess, then fry in the hot oil, turning every 1–2 minutes, until golden brown.

3 Dust the fritters with icing sugar and serve hot with a scoop of dairy-free or soya ice cream (not cow's milk though, as it's not allowed on the low FODMAP diet).

Preparation time: 15 minutes
Cooking time: 10 minutes
Serves: 4

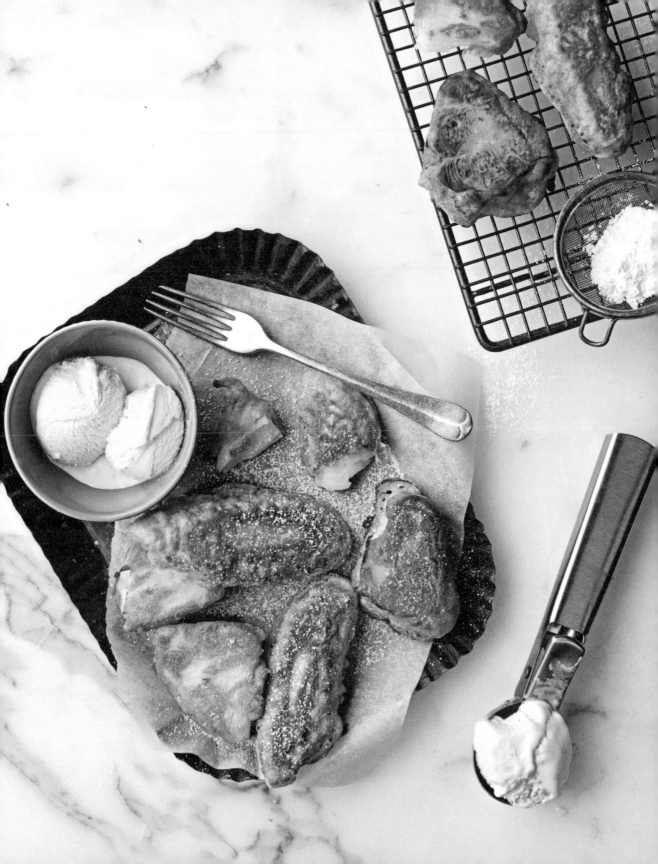

Almond Macaroons

These chewy macaroons keep for four days in an airtight container at room temperature. They are best served with stewed fruit or a mug of tea. **Remember, almonds need to be portion controlled to 10 nuts/10g per serving, so stick to two or three biscuits only per sitting.**

 Portion size: 14g **Kcals:** 65 **Fat:** 3.9g **Saturated fat:** 0.3g **Carbs:** 5.1g **Sugar:** 4.6g **Fibre:** 1.2g **Protein:** 1.8g **Salt:** 0.01g
Allergens: Tree nuts, eggs

INGREDIENTS

100g whole almonds (preferably blanched)
65g granulated sugar
1 large egg white
⅓ tsp almond or vanilla extract
pinch of salt
icing sugar, for dusting
15g flaked almonds, for decorating

WHAT TO DO

1 Preheat the oven to 175°C. Line a baking sheet with non-stick baking paper and spray with oil or grease with butter.
2 Blend the whole almonds and the granulated sugar in a food processor until they are finely ground. Add the egg white, almond or vanilla extract and a pinch salt and blend again until combined.
3 Roll the mixture into small balls about 2.5cm in diameter and arrange on the prepared baking sheet spaced about 5cm apart. Slightly flatten the balls and dust lightly with icing sugar. Gently press some almond slices into each macaroon.
4 Bake in the middle rack of the oven for 10–15 minutes, until the macaroons are starting to turn golden. Cool on a wire rack.

Preparation time: 15 minutes
Cooking time: 10–15 minutes
Makes: 16

Coconut and Chia Rice Pudding

A creamy, sticky, delicious, healthy pudding. It's the ideal snack post-training or it can also be used as a meal replacement (just be aware of the high kcal content!). **Remember to portion control your coconut milk to <125ml per serving** (the dairy substitute, not the can of coconut milk used in cooking).

 Portion size: 293g **Kcals:** 193 **Fat:** 4.3g **Saturated fat:** 4.3g **Carbs:** 34.5g **Sugar:** 8.3g **Fibre:** 2.4g **Protein:** 3g **Salt:** 0.1g
Allergens: May contain sulphites

WHAT TO DO

1 Place the rice, water, coconut milk, sugar, chia seeds and coconut essence in a deep pot. Stir well and slowly bring to the boil, then reduce the heat and simmer very gently for 20–30 minutes, stirring every now and then, until all the liquid has been absorbed and the rice is just cooked.
2 Spoon the cooked rice pudding into a serving dish and sprinkle with desiccated coconut before serving.

INGREDIENTS

130g pudding rice
500ml water
500ml coconut milk
2 tbsp caster sugar
2 tbsp chia seeds
½ tsp coconut essence
dessicated coconut, to serve

Preparation time: 10 minutes
Cooking time: 40 minutes
Serves: 4

Lemon and Lime Mini Cheesecakes

You can use almond flour or ground almonds to make the cheesecake crust (recommended serving is <24g per portion). You are safe if you keep to one mini cheesecake per sitting – the reason why these are pre-portioned!

Portion size: 58g **Kcals:** 184 **Fat:** 13.9g **Saturated fat:** 6.1g **Carbs:** 10.6g **Sugar:** 7g **Fibre:** 1.2g **Protein:** 3.9g **Salt:** 0.3g
Allergens: Tree nuts, eggs, milk, may contain gluten

INGREDIENTS

For the base:
60g butter, diced
60g/about 6 oatcakes
60g almond flour or ground almonds
20g/12 macadamia nuts
2 tbsp maple syrup

For the filling:
200g lactose-free cream cheese
50g caster sugar
1 tsp vanilla extract
2 medium eggs
zest and juice of 1 lemon
zest and juice of 1 lime

WHAT TO DO

1 Preheat the oven to 150°C. Lightly grease 2 x 6-hole silicone muffin trays.

2 To make the base, blend the butter, oatcakes, almond flour, nuts and maple syrup until well combined. Divide between the muffin trays and press down with a shot glass until the base is flat. Bake in the oven for 10 minutes, then cool on a wire rack.

3 Meanwhile, make the cheesecake filling by blending the cream cheese, sugar and vanilla extract until smooth. Add the eggs and blend again. Squeeze the lemon and lime juice into the cheesecake filling, followed by the lemon and lime zest. Gently mix together.

4 Spoon the filling onto the bases. You can tap the tray gently on the worktop to get a more even surface and get rid of any air bubbles.

5 Bake for 15–20 minutes, until the filling has set. Cool on a wire rack for 1–2 hours before serving or chill in the fridge to make them cool faster if you just can't wait!

Preparation time: 20 minutes
Cooking time: 30 minutes
Makes: 12

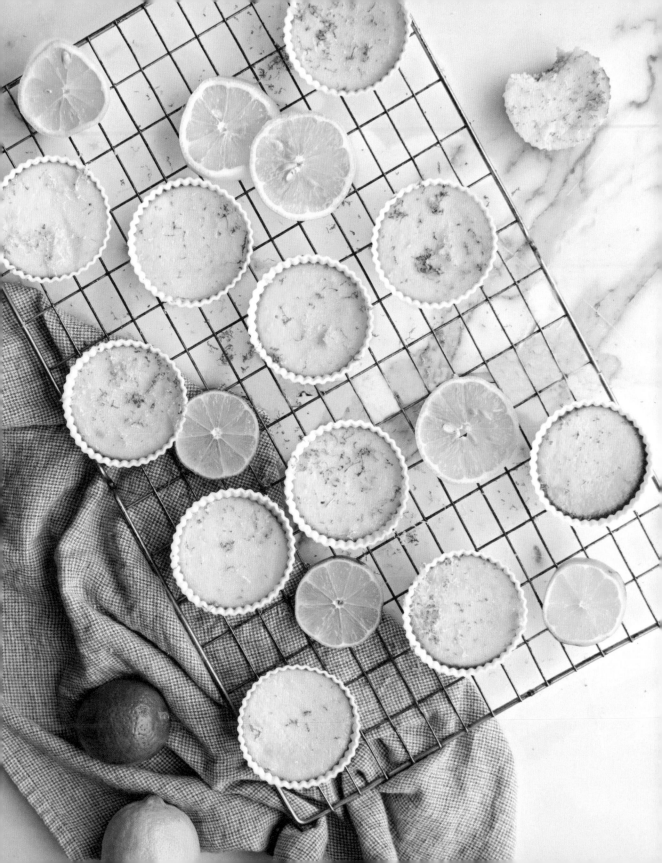

Friendly Chocolate Truffles

These truffles are so simple to make, yet so divine … mmmm! **You can get away with using normal low-fat cream cheese or quark in this recipe if you keep to a normal portion (a maximum of two truffles per sitting). Remember to keep to a maximum serving of 18g desiccated coconut at a time.**

Portion size: 18g **Kcals:** 81 **Fat:** 6.2g **Saturated fat:** 4g **Carbs:** 4.6g **Sugar:** 4g **Fibre:** 1.2g **Protein:** 1.1g
Salt: 0.04g **Allergens:** Milk, may contain eggs, may contain sesame, may contain sulphites, may contain nuts

INGREDIENTS

50g lactose-free soft cheese spread,
    e.g. cream cheese or quark
2 tbsp maple syrup
100g dark chocolate
20g desiccated coconut, for rolling

WHAT TO DO

1 Beat the soft cheese and maple syrup in a bowl or food processor until smooth.
2 Break the chocolate into small pieces and melt in a heatproof bowl set above a pan of simmering water. Add the melted chocolate to the cheese mixture and stir to combine. Chill in the fridge for about 1 hour, until the chocolate is hard enough to roll it.
3 Using a teaspoon, scoop out the mixture and roll into small balls between the palms of your hands. Place the coconut on a plate, then roll the balls in it until they are evenly coated.
4 Kept in a jar in the fridge, these truffles will last for up to three days.

Preparation time: 10 minutes
Cooking time: 1 hour chilling time
Makes: 12

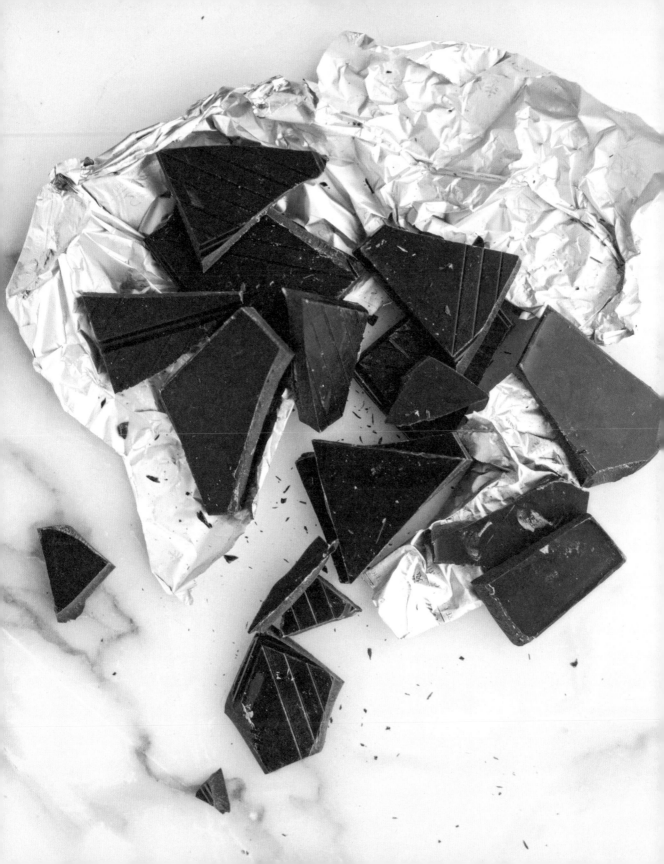

Chocolate Ice Cream

This is a healthy, low-calorie ice cream, but it tastes amazing! **Do make sure you keep to the chocolate soya milk portion of 60ml at a time, so this recipe is fine if you stick to one portion.**

Portion size: 107g **Kcals:** 210 **Fat:** 12.6g **Saturated fat:** 5g **Carbs:** 16.6g **Sugar:** 14g **Fibre:** 3.1g **Protein:** 5.4g **Salt:** 0.2g
Allergens: Peanuts, soya, may contain milk, may contain nuts

INGREDIENTS

200g/2 bananas, frozen
50g smooth peanut butter
125ml chocolate soya milk
50g dark chocolate chips
a few fresh mint leaves, to decorate

WHAT TO DO

1 Blend the frozen bananas, peanut butter and chocolate soya milk together.
2 Stir in the chocolate chips before placing in a lidded container in the freezer for 3 hours.
3 Serve with fresh mint leaves.

Preparation time: 10 minutes
Cooking time: 3+ hours in the freezer
Serves: 4

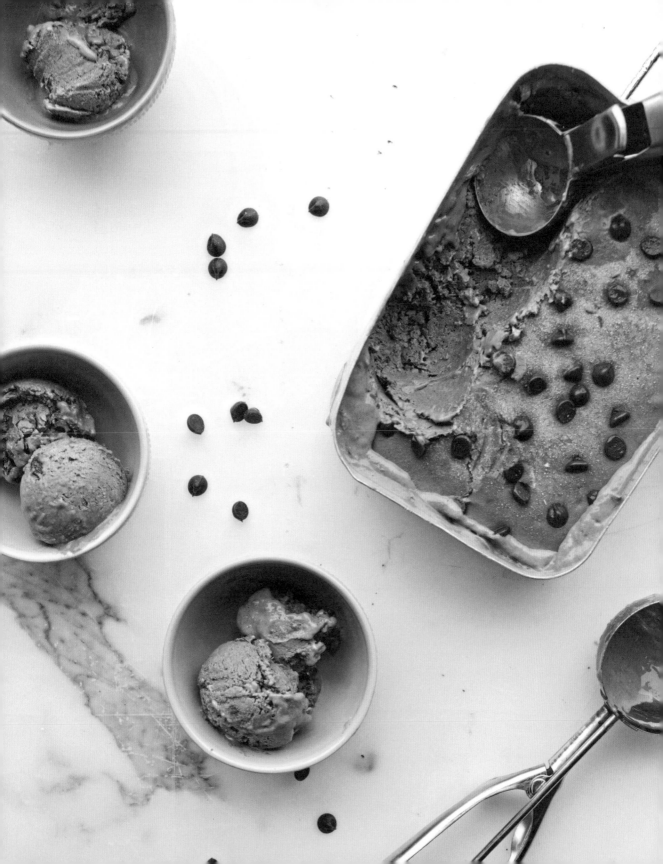

Snacks

Avoid unhealthy temptations from petrol stations, cafés and vending machines by keeping a stash of **nutritious** low FODMAP **snacks** to hand. The following recipes are snacks that need little or no preparation and will tide you over until your next meal. Some of the recipes in this chapter, like the **sweet** and **spicy** nuts and blueberry muffins, are great for eating on the go if you have a busy day.

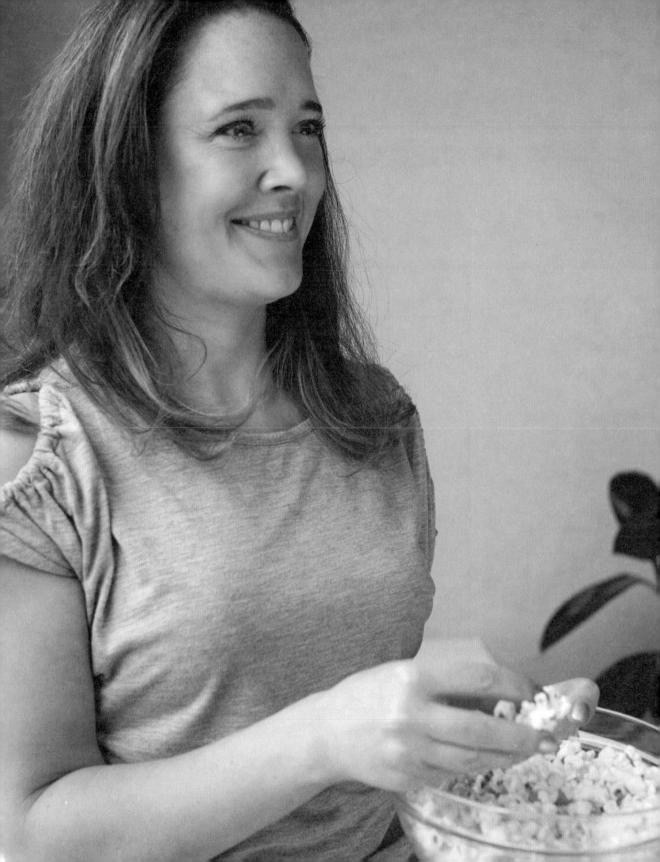

Frozen Banana Bites

These will help fix a sweet craving in a flash! **Be sure to keep almond butter to a maximum of 12g per sitting (approx. two bites).**

Portion size: 28g **Kcals:** 66 **Fat:** 4g **Saturated fat:** 1g **Carbs:** 5.1g **Sugar:** 4.4g **Fibre:** 1.4g **Protein:** 1.5g **Salt:** 0.1g
Allergens: Tree nuts, may contain milk

INGREDIENTS

200g/2 bananas
50g almond butter
30g dark chocolate

WHAT TO DO

1 Peel and slice the bananas into 1cm-thick slices (approx. 10 slices per banana). Place some almond butter on a banana slice and place another slice of banana on top, like a sandwich.
2 Place a lollipop stick or toothpick through the 'sandwich' and place in the freezer for 1 hour. When the banana is frozen, remove it from the freezer.
3 Place the chocolate in a microwave-safe bowl and melt. Swirl each banana lolly in the chocolate until it is completely coated. Freeze again until the chocolate sets, about 1 hour more.
4 Keep in the freezer until required.

Preparation time: 10 minutes
Cooking time: 2 hours in the freezer
Makes: 10

Melon and Feta Skewers

This refreshing yet nutritious snack is a perfect balance of sweetness, saltiness and crunch!

Portion size: 104g **Kcals:** 115 **Fat:** 7.6g **Saturated fat:** 3.8g
Carbs: 5.3g **Sugar:** 4.2g **Fibre:** 1.9g **Protein:** 5.3g **Salt:** 0.7g
Allergens: Milk

INGREDIENTS

260g/ ½ melon, cut into chunks
100g feta, cut into cubes
2 tbsp poppy seeds
6–8 black olives
juice of 1 lime

WHAT TO DO

1 Put the melon and feta on separate plates and sprinkle with poppy seeds. Gently toss until the seeds stick.
2 Thread a cube of melon followed by cube of feta onto three or four long skewers. Stick an olive at each end.
3 Arrange on a platter and squeeze over the lime juice. Chill for 30 minutes before serving.

Preparation time: 10 minutes
Cooking time: 30 minutes in the fridge
Serves: 4

Strawberry and Lime Sorbet

A tangy and refreshing sorbet that's ice cream's nearest competitor!

Portion size: 243g **Kcals:** 57 **Fat:** 0.7g **Saturated fat:** 0.1g
Carbs: 10.8g **Salt:** 0.04g **Fibre:** 2.6g **Protein:** 0.6g
Sugar: 10g **Allergens:** May contain soya, may contain tree nuts depending on type of milk used

INGREDIENTS

125g strawberries
240ml water
60ml soya or almond milk
juice of 1 lime
1 tbsp maple syrup

WHAT TO DO

1 Blend all the ingredients together until smooth. Place in an airtight container and freeze for at least 3 hours or overnight.
2 Blend again just before serving.

Preparation time: 10 minutes
Cooking time: Minimum 3 hours in the freezer
Serves: 2

Kale Chips

The healthy crisp! Perfect for sharing with friends at a party or in front of the TV. Kale is a leafy green vegetable that's allowed on a low FODMAP diet.

Portion size: 43g **Kcals:** 102 **Fat:** 9.7g **Saturated fat:** 1.5g **Carbs:** 0.9g **Sugar:** 0.8g **Fibre:** 1.5g **Protein:** 2.1g **Salt:** 0.7g
Allergens: Gluten, sesame, soya

INGREDIENTS

50g kale (after removing stems)
1 tbsp sesame oil or olive oil
2 tsp low-sodium soya sauce
1 tbsp sesame seeds

WHAT TO DO

1 Preheat the oven to 175°C.
2 Wash the kale leaves that have been stripped from their stems, then dry thoroughly in kitchen paper or a clean tea towel (otherwise the chips will be soggy). Tear the kale into large pieces and place them in a bowl.
3 Add the oil, soya sauce and sesame seeds and toss all the ingredients together with your hands. Try to make sure all the kale is covered in oil.
4 Spread the kale out flat on one or two baking sheets. Bake in the oven for 6–7 minutes. They are ready before they've completely crisped up – you'll notice that they will still be soft in the middle.
5 Eat immediately!

Preparation time: 10 minutes
Cooking time: 10 minutes
Serves: 2

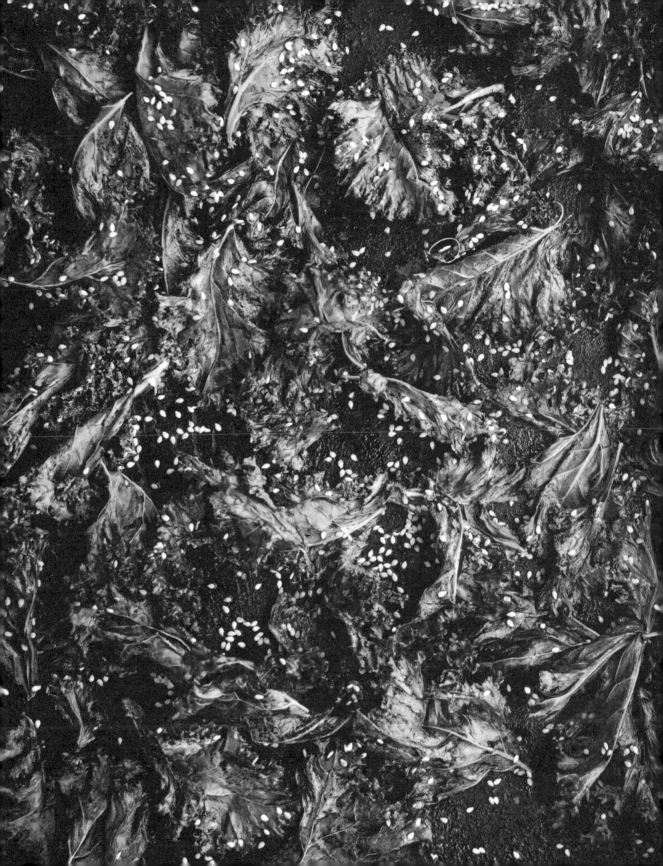

Dark Chocolate Oat Clusters

These are great when you're feeling extra hungry between meals or as an on-the-go snack. **Remember, only 13g dried cranberries and 12g almond butter are allowed at any one time. You will get away with two of these cluster portions at a time to keep within the recommended amount.**

Portion size: 22g **Kcals:** 85 **Fat:** 5.3g **Saturated fat:** 1.6g **Carbs:** 6.1g **Sugar:** 3.2g **Fibre:** 1.7g **Protein:** 2g **Salt:** 0.1g
Allergens: Soya, tree nuts, may contain milk, may contain gluten, may contain sulphites

INGREDIENTS
70g almond butter
70g dark chocolate
3 tbsp almond milk
78g dried cranberries
50g oats, preferably jumbo oats
1 tsp vanilla extract

WHAT TO DO
1 Place the almond butter, chocolate and almond milk in a saucepan. Cook over a low heat for about 3 minutes, until everything has melted together. Stir in the dried cranberries, oats and vanilla extract and remove from the heat.
2 Divide into about 12 portions by putting spoonfuls of the mixture into mini cupcake cases or directly onto a baking tray lined with non-stick baking paper. Place in the fridge to set for at least 10 minutes before serving.

Preparation time: 5 minutes
Cooking time: 15 minutes
Makes: 12

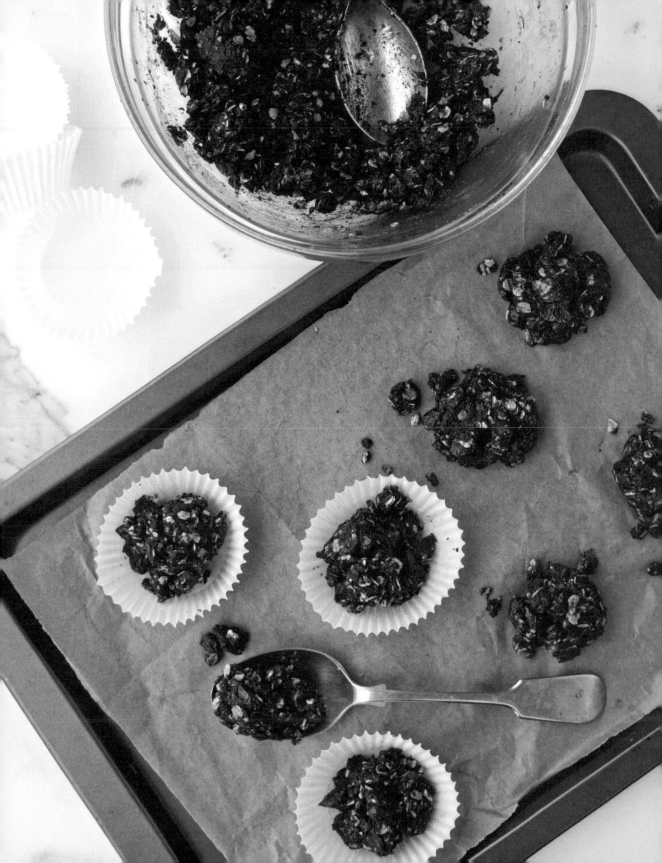

Black Pepper Oat Crackers

These are really tasty just as they are, but you could replace the black pepper with flaxseeds, sesame seeds or sunflower seeds for variety. These crackers keep well in an airtight container and are great for the lunchbox. Oats are a brilliant source of soluble fibre and beta-glucans and are known to help those who suffer with constipation and bloating.

Portion size: 10g **Kcals:** 34 **Fat:** 1.7g **Saturated fat:** 0.3g **Carbs:** 3.9g **Sugar:** 0.02g **Fibre:** 0.5g **Protein:** 0.7g **Salt:** 0.1g
Allergens: May contain gluten

INGREDIENTS

180g oats
2 tsp freshly ground black pepper
½ tsp salt
1/8 tsp baking soda
3 tbsp olive oil
60–100ml hot water

WHAT TO DO

1 Preheat the oven to 180°C. Line two baking trays with non-stick baking paper and stick it to the trays with a little oil or butter.
2 Grind the oats into a fine powder in a food processor. Add the pepper, salt and baking soda and mix thoroughly.
3 In a large bowl, whisk the oil and about 60ml of hot water together and slowly add the oat mix. Add more water if needed for the dough to form a ball.
4 Divide the dough in half and place on the two lined baking trays. Roll out thinly – the thinner, the better, and not more than 5mm thick. Divide into cracker shapes with a pizza cutter or a sharp knife.
5 Bake for about 20 minutes, until browned. Allow to cool on a wire rack, then store in an airtight container.

Preparation time: 20 minutes
Cooking time: 20 minutes
Makes: 30 crackers

Blueberry and Linseed Muffins

These are a tasty and filling snack but could also be used for breakfast. They freeze well too – wrap each muffin individually and take one out of the freezer when needed for a handy snack on the run. Use these to boost your daily fibre intake.

Portion size: 86g **Kcals:** 199 **Fat:** 7.3g **Saturated fat:** 1.5g **Carbs:** 23g **Sugar:** 7.6g **Fibre:** 5g **Protein:** 7.1g **Salt:** 0.2g
Allergens: Eggs, milk, may contain gluten, may contain sulphites

WHAT TO DO

1 Preheat the oven to 180°C.
2 Line two muffin tins with silicone muffin cases. Spray the muffin cases with spray oil or grease with a pastry brush dipped in oil.
3 Mash the banana with a fork. Add the eggs, maple syrup, oil and vanilla extract and mix well.
4 In another bowl, combine the oat flour, linseeds, oat bran and baking powder together. Pour the banana mixture into the flour mix and fold in with a spatula until combined. Add the yogurt and then the milk and stir until the batter is moist but not too runny. Finally, gently fold in the blueberries and lemon zest.
5 Spoon the batter into the muffin cases. Bake in the oven for 18–20 minutes, until firm to the touch.

INGREDIENTS

100g/1 ripe banana, mashed
2 eggs
2 tbsp maple syrup
2 tsp olive oil
1 tsp vanilla extract
250g oat flour (blend normal oats to a fine consistency to make flour)
70g ground linseeds
40g oat bran
1 tsp baking powder
125g cow's milk natural yogurt
120ml lactose-free milk
125g blueberries
zest of 1 lemon

Preparation time: 15 minutes
Cooking time: 20 minutes
Makes: 12 muffins

Nut and Seed Balls

These are particularly moreish, but **only two or three per sitting is recommended**. Nuts and seeds are a trendy, nutritious snack. They are great sources of essential fats, fibre and protein. **If you decide to choose almonds or hazelnuts, remember that only 10 of either nut is recommended at any one sitting.**

Portion size: 20g **Kcals:** 81 **Fat:** 5.8g **Saturated fat:** 1.5g **Carbs:** 4.2g **Sugar:** 1.8g **Fibre:** 0.7g **Protein:** 2.8g **Salt:** 0.01g
Allergens: Tree nuts, milk, sesame, may contain peanuts, may contain gluten, may contain sulphites

INGREDIENTS

100g low FODMAP mixed nuts
    (e.g. walnuts, Brazil nuts, pecans,
    macadamias)
100g mixed seeds (e.g. sunflower,
    pumpkin, sesame)
40g oats
100g Greek yogurt
2 tbsp maple syrup
1 tsp ground cinnamon
1 tsp vanilla extract
1 tbsp desiccated coconut, for rolling

WHAT TO DO

1 Put the nuts and seeds in a food processor and blend until coarse. Add the oats and blend again. Add the yogurt, maple syrup, cinnamon and vanilla extract and blend thoroughly. The mixture should combine to form balls easily. Roll the mixture into balls approximately the size of a walnut.

2 Spread the desiccated coconut on a flat plate and roll the balls in it to cover them. Place in the freezer for 1 hour before eating.

3 These can be eaten frozen or stored in the fridge for up to four days.

Preparation time: 20 minutes
Cooking time: 1 hour in the freezer
Makes: 20 balls

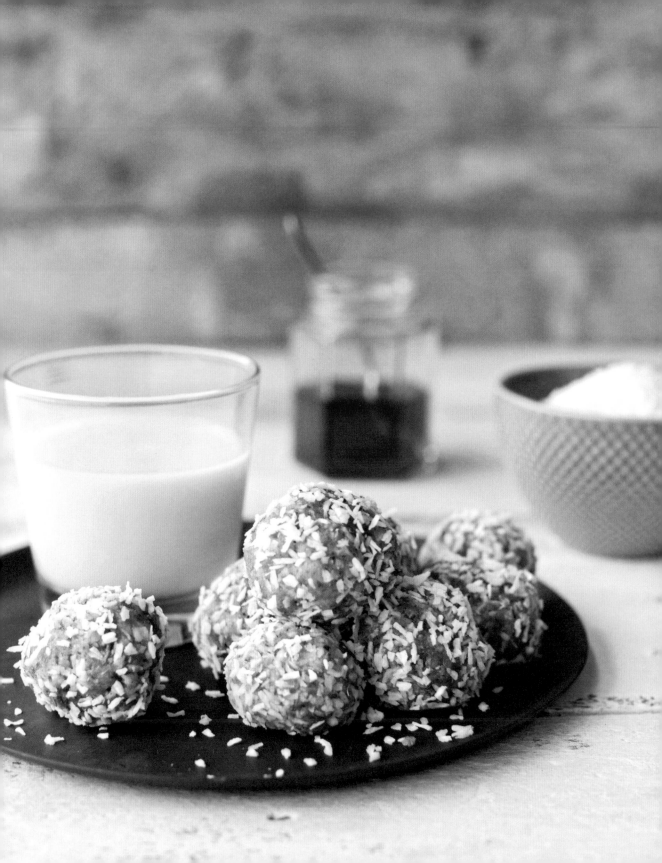

Parmesan Popcorn

Made for sharing! A snack that's a good source of fibre, low calorie and filling. Air-popped popcorn is best for this recipe, but heating 1 teaspoon of oil in a pan and adding the popcorn kernels works just as well.

Portion size: 38g **Kcals:** 147 **Fat:** 3.6g **Saturated fat:** 1.6g **Carbs:** 20g **Sugar:** 0.3g **Fibre:** 4.2g **Protein:** 6.4g **Salt:** 0.1g
Allergens: Milk

INGREDIENTS

120g popcorn kernels
1 tsp olive oil (optional)
30g grated Parmesan
2 tsp dried thyme
salt and freshly ground black pepper

WHAT TO DO

1 Air-pop the popcorn or heat 1 teaspoon of oil in heavy-bottomed saucepan set over a medium heat and add the popcorn kernels. Cook with the lid on, shaking occasionally, until all the kernels have popped.
2 Sprinkle the hot popcorn with the grated Parmesan and toss until well coated, then add the thyme. Season and serve immediately.

Preparation time: 5 minutes
Cooking time: 5 minutes
Serves: 4

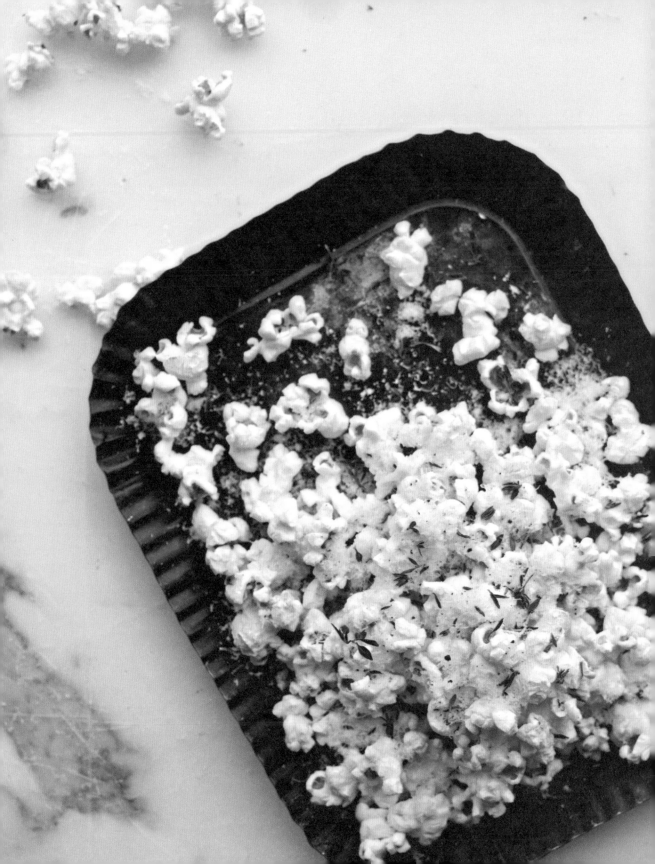

Sweet and Spicy Nuts

Nuts should be a part of your daily and habitual diets. This recipe is a fancy way to eat some more and is great for get-togethers, holidays or movie nights. **Remember, a portion of nuts is about 36g mixed nuts, so only take a maximum one-third of these nuts at a time. If you stick to one portion, you will be safe.**

Serving: 32g **Kcals:** 188 **Fat:** 16.5g **Saturated fat:** 1.7g **Carbs:** 5.1g **Sugar:** 3.6g **Fibre:** 2.2g **Protein:** 4g
Salt: 0.04g **Allergens:** Tree nuts

INGREDIENTS

50g pecans
50g walnuts
24g almonds
30g pumpkin seeds
2 tsp maple syrup
1 tsp olive oil
1 tbsp chopped fresh rosemary leaves
½ tsp smoked paprika
pinch of salt

WHAT TO DO

1 Preheat the oven to 180°C.
2 Toss the nuts, pumpkin seeds, maple syrup, oil, rosemary, paprika and salt together in a medium bowl and coat the nuts evenly.
3 Transfer to a baking sheet and bake, tossing occasionally, for 20–25 minutes, until the nuts are toasted and the maple syrup has caramelised.
4 Transfer to a sheet of parchment paper and spread out in an even layer to prevent clusters from forming. Cool before serving and share!

Preparation time: 10 minutes
Cooking time: 25 minutes
Serves: 6

Banana Biccies

You can vary the texture of these delicious banana biccies by using different types of ground or steel-cut oats and adding 20g of crushed walnuts or pecans instead of the seeds.

 Portion size: 42g **Kcals:** 91 **Fat:** 1.4g **Saturated fat:** 0.2g **Carbs:** 17.1g **Sugar:** 9.3g **Fibre:** 1.8g **Protein:** 1.7g
Salt: 0.1g **Allergens:** May contain gluten, may contain sesame

WHAT TO DO

1 Preheat the oven to 180°C. Lightly grease a baking tray.
2 Mash the bananas in a bowl with a fork until smooth, then stir in the oats until fully mixed. Allow to stand for 5 minutes, then add all the remaining ingredients and mix well. If you've used pinhead oats, the mixture may look watery.
3 Put heaped tablespoons of the mixture onto the greased baking tray spaced about 8cm apart.
4 Bake in the oven for 20–25 minutes, until golden brown and firm to the touch in the centre. Cool on a wire rack before eating.

INGREDIENTS

240g/2 large very ripe bananas
80g pinhead or porridge oats
50g light brown sugar
20g mixed seeds (e.g. sunflower, chia, linseeds)
1 tbsp cornflour
1 tsp baking powder
1 tsp ground cinnamon
½ tsp ground nutmeg

Preparation time: 10 minutes
Cooking time: 25 minutes
Makes: 10

Drinks, Juices & Smoothies

While a drink of water (whether plain or adorned with a *citrus* slice or sprig of mint) is the perfect no-calorie beverage, not everyone finds it easy to drink all of the time. We've included some low FODMAP-friendly beverages, both *hot* and *cold*, to whet your appetite and leave your taste buds *zinging*.

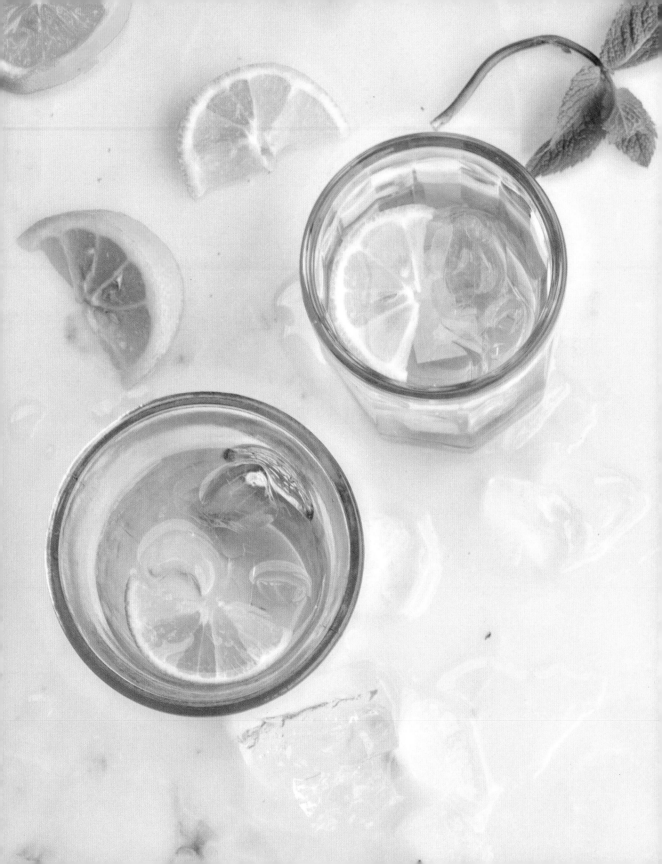

How to stay hydrated

Water is a fundamental and essential part of the body. It has varied functions, including transporting nutrients in the blood, removing waste products excreted in the urine and acting as a lubricant and shock absorber in our joints.

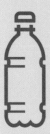

Thirst is the body's way of indicating a need for water or fluid. Dehydration can slow us down and even alters our metabolism in a bid to conserve energy. Even slight dehydration can leave you tired and sluggish. It can also result in:

* Delayed reaction time
* Headache or foggy thinking
* Constipation
* Irritability
* Nausea or dizziness
* Poor concentration
* Reduced muscular strength and physical endurance

It's especially important that you stay fully hydrated on the low FODMAP diet. Your needs will vary depending on your body size and activity levels, but most of us need between 1.5 and 3 litres of fluid a day.

* Stick to water whenever possible, but avoid coconut water.
* Limit caffeinated beverages (like coffee) and find your tolerance level. For many people this is one or two cups per day. Try the full aroma and flavour of a good decaffeinated coffee instead.
* Avoid caffeinated energy drinks such as Red Bull, Monster and Energise Edge.
* Tea, particularly weak tea, contains half the caffeine levels of some coffees.
* Drink peppermint tea, green tea, red tea or white tea. Avoid chicory, fennel, chamomile and chai teas.
* Avoid fizzy drinks and carbonated water, as they can often make symptoms worse.
* Keep to the recommended limits for alcohol and avoid binge drinking.

It's always nice to try something different. Enjoy some of these tasty alternatives when the occasion allows.

Green Tea Latte

You can use green tea or matcha powder to make this cooling drink.

Portion size: 258ml **Kcals:** 93 **Fat:** 2.5g **Saturated fat:** 1.5g **Carbs:** 9g **Sugar:** 8.8g **Fibre:** 0.3g **Protein:** 8.5 **Salt:** 0.3g
Allergens: Milk

WHAT TO DO

1 Put the milk and tea bags or powder in a saucepan and bring to the boil, then reduce the heat and simmer for 1–2 minutes.
2 Strain out the tea bags and sweeten with the maple syrup, if using. Serve hot with a sprinkle of cinnamon on top.

INGREDIENTS

500ml lactose-free milk
2 green tea bags or 2 tsp matcha powder
1 tsp maple syrup (optional)
pinch of ground cinnamon

Preparation time: 2 minutes
Cooking time: 5 minutes
Serves: 2

Peanut Butter, Oat and Banana Milkshake

This is a good choice if you need to run out the door and eat your breakfast on the way! It's also an excellent post-workout drink. If you can, cut the banana into slices and freeze them ahead of time to give your smoothie a lovely ice cream-like texture.

Portion size: 330ml **Kcals:** 251 **Fat:** 11g **Saturated fat:** 2.5g **Carbs:** 26g **Sugar:** 17.6g **Fibre:** 7.8g **Protein:** 7.4g **Salt:** 0.4g
Allergens: Milk, peanuts, tree nuts, may contain gluten

INGREDIENTS

500ml almond milk or
    lactose-free milk
100g/1 medium banana, chopped
30g peanut butter
20g oats
1 tbsp ground linseeds or
    any other seeds

WHAT TO DO

1 Put all the ingredients into a blender and blend until really smooth. Pour into a tall glass and serve immediately.

Preparation time: 5 minutes
Cooking time: N/A
Serves: 2

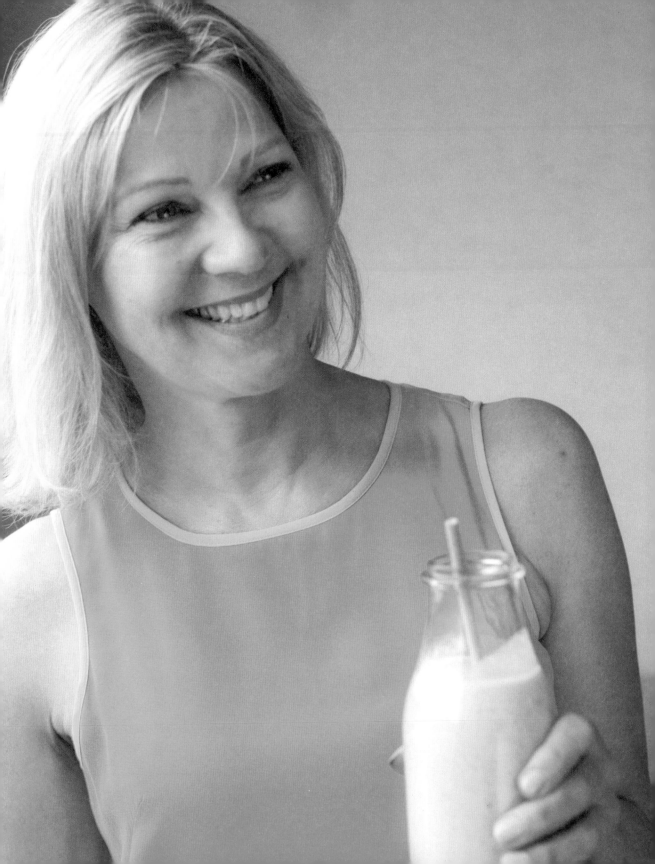

Antioxidant Soothing Slushie

This drink contains peppermint, which has been known to help soothe a troubled tummy.
The ideal portion is 200ml.

Portion size: 200ml **Kcals:** 49 **Fat:** 0.5g **Saturated fat:** 0.03g **Carbs:** 8.7g **Sugar:** 8.4g **Fibre:** 3g **Protein:** 0.9g **Salt:** 0.01g
Allergens: None

INGREDIENTS
250ml peppermint tea (cold)
100g strawberries
60g/1 kiwi
50g blueberries
50g/about 5 ice cubes

WHAT TO DO
1 Put all the ingredients into a blender and blend until really smooth. Pour into a tall glass and serve immediately.

Preparation time: 5 minutes
Cooking time: N/A
Serves: 2

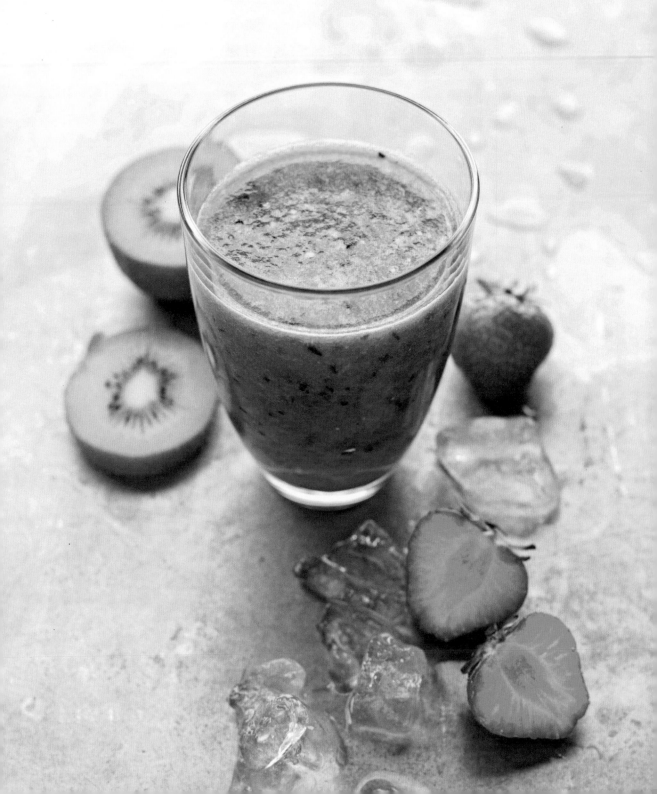

Tropical Green Smoothie

This smoothie will surprise you in many ways. Close your eyes and think piña colada!
The recommended portion size is 200ml.

Portion size: 200ml **Kcals:** 86 **Fat:** 2.1g **Saturated fat:** 1.7g **Carbs:** 14.2g **Sugar:** 13.2g **Fibre:** 1.5g **Protein:** 1.8g **Salt:** 0.1g
Allergens: None

INGREDIENTS

180g pineapple chunks

160g spinach

120g/1 large ripe banana, peeled
(previously frozen in chunks if
possible)

350ml coconut milk

1 tsp vanilla extract

WHAT TO DO

1 Place all the ingredients in a blender and blend until smooth.
Pour into a tall glass and serve chilled (the frozen ingredients
will instantly chill this drink).

Preparation time: 5 minutes
Cooking time: N/A
Serves: 4

Cucumber Juice Drink

If you find it difficult to drink water, keep a jug of this in the fridge and sip it throughout the day to help meet your fluid requirements.

Portion size: 200ml **Kcals:** 13.6 **Fat:** 0.5g **Saturated fat:** 0g **Carbs:** 1.2g **Sugar:** 0.9g **Fibre:** 0.6g **Protein:** 0.8g **Salt:** 0.01g
Allergens: None

WHAT TO DO
1 Blend all the ingredients together in a blender, then strain through a fine-mesh sieve. Serve chilled or on ice.

INGREDIENTS
600g/1 cucumber, peeled and seeds scraped out
5 cardamom pods
1cm piece of fresh ginger or to taste (small amount!)
1 litre water
½ tsp lemon juice, or to taste

Preparation time: 5 minutes
Cooking time: N/A
Serves: 8

Almond Milk

It's pretty easy to make your own almond milk at home. Make sure to buy the almonds without their skins. Some people like to add 1 tablespoon of maple syrup to this recipe to sweeten it, but we prefer cinnamon to give it some warmth. **You can enjoy 100ml of homemade almond milk as a serving, but remember that if you want to eat whole raw almonds, you need to limit the serving size to 10 nuts. However, shop-bought almond milk is low FODMAP up to 250ml per serving.**

Portion size: 59ml **Kcals:** 80 **Fat:** 6.9g **Saturated:** 6.5g **Carbs:** 0.8g **Sugar:** 0.5g **Fibre:** 1.9g **Protein:** 2.6g **Salt:** 0.01g **Allergens:** Tree nuts

INGREDIENTS

100g almonds, without skins
300ml water
2 tsp ground cinnamon

WHAT TO DO

1 Soak the almonds overnight (or for at least 6 hours) to soften them.
2 Drain the almonds and blend with the water and cinnamon until you get a smooth, milky consistency.
3 Strain through a fine-mesh sieve or a flexible plastic sieve to remove any remaining skins or lumps. Store in an airtight container in the fridge for up to seven days.

Preparation time: 10 minutes (excluding soaking time)
Cooking time: N/A
Serves: 6

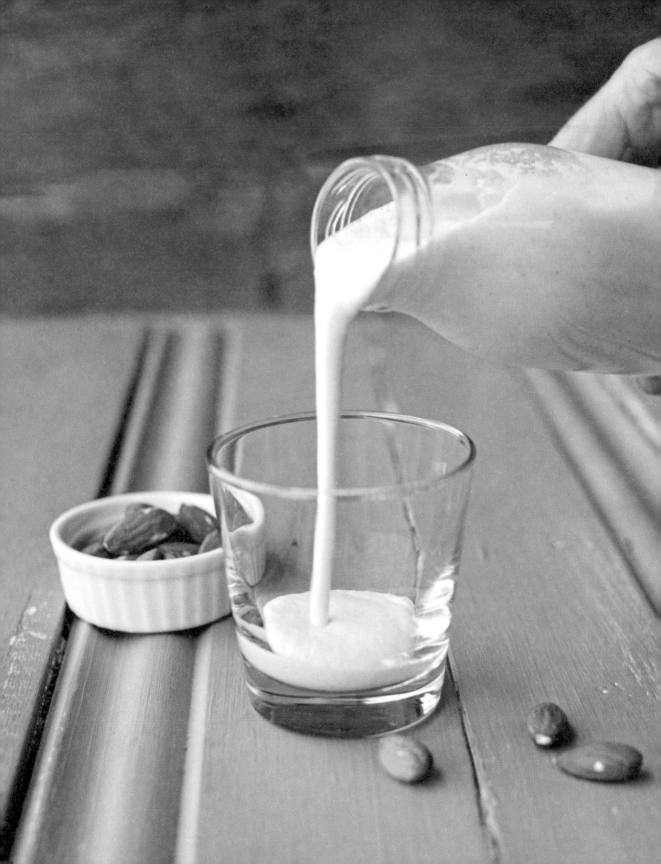

Yogi Tea

This tea originally started as part of traditional Indian medicine, where the spices were intended to be healing and nourishing. The mix of cardamom, ginger, cinnamon and cloves is delightful. Whether you are recovering from a workout, catching up with friends or just want to warm up on a cold day, this is the perfect tea for every occasion.

 Portion size: 320ml **Kcals:** 35 **Fat:** 1.7g **Saturated fat:** 0.3g **Carbs:** 2g **Sugar:** 0.2g **Fibre:** 1.7g **Protein:** 2.4g **Salt:** 0.01g **Allergens:** May contain milk, soya

INGREDIENTS

20 green cardamom pods, crushed slightly
15 whole cloves
15 black peppercorns
5 x 5cm cinnamon sticks
8cm piece of fresh ginger
1.8 litres water
700ml soya or rice milk (optional)
½ tsp black tea leaves
maple syrup, to taste (optional)

WHAT TO DO

1 Place the cardamom pods, cloves, peppercorns, cinnamon sticks, ginger and water in a saucepan and bring to the boil. Reduce the heat and simmer gently, covered, for 30–40 minutes. Add more water if it evaporates.

2 Add the milk, if using, and the black tea. Bring to the boil again, then immediately remove from the heat. Add maple syrup to taste, strain through a fine-mesh sieve and serve.

3 This can be stored in the fridge for up to one week if you've used milk, or longer for clear tea.

Preparation time: 10 minutes
Cooking time: 45 minutes
Serves: 6–12

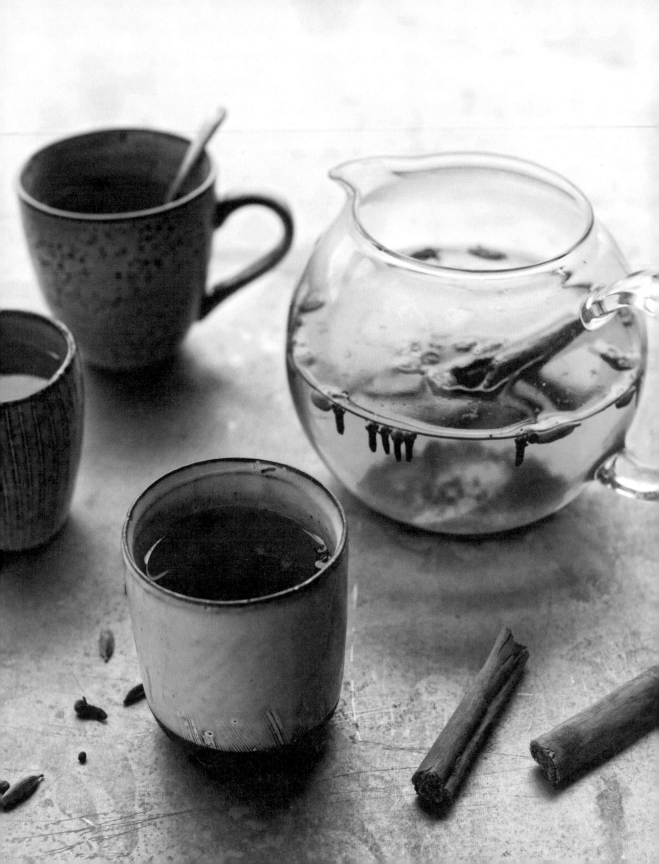

Appendix

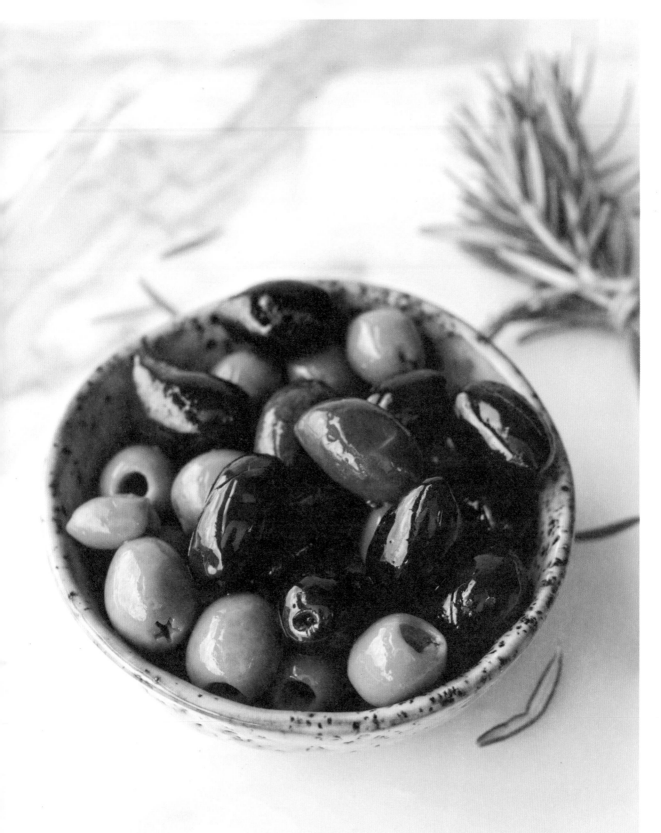

Gut sensitivities in digestive disorders: A brief insight and tips to manage it

Irritable bowel syndrome (IBS)

People with IBS have a hypersensitive gut, meaning the nerve endings around the intestine are very sensitive. Symptoms come and go over the long term. There are many symptoms and permutations and we can't go into all of them here, but the most common symptoms include bloating and/or distension, tummy discomfort or abdominal pain, excessive wind, constipation and/or diarrhoea.

You can monitor the severity of your IBS symptoms before and after the first stage of the low FODMAP diet. We have included a questionnaire (see the symptom assessment on page 208) to help you. You can discuss the results with your dietitian or GP and track your symptoms over time.

Causes of IBS

The actual cause of IBS is still unknown, but certain factors are thought to trigger symptoms. These include:

* An initial bout of gastritis or a gut infection may precede the initial symptoms.
* An imbalance or overgrowth of bacteria in the small intestine.
* High stress and anxiety levels (see pages 200–202 for more on the gut–brain connection).
* While FODMAPs are not the cause of IBS, restricting them reduces symptoms.

There's a bewildering array of expensive supplements, medications and miracle diets offering magical cures and the devil knows what else to IBS patients. But just as you would research the market before buying a car or a house, you should also look at the evidence for a treatment or a diet rather than blindly following the latest fad or craze.

Diagnosing IBS

Your GP will assess your symptoms and make a diagnosis on the basis of your medical and dietary history. Blood tests are required to rule out other digestive conditions with similar symptoms. You may be referred to a gastroenterologist for further investigation and to rule out other disorders, such as inflammatory bowel disease or coeliac disease.

Managing IBS

Draw up a suitable management plan with the help of your doctor or dietitian, which may include:

* The low FODMAP diet (see the low FODMAP stages on pages 6–10)
* Probiotic treatment (see the section on the microbiome on pages 202–204)
* Pharmaceutical therapy (anti-spasmodic, anti-diarrhoeal, laxatives)
* Psychological therapy (mindfulness, relaxation treatments, yoga, CBT, counselling) (see the section on mindfulness on pages 201–202)

Dietary changes

Dietary changes can significantly improve IBS symptoms. You should try these first before commencing a low FODMAP diet.

* Eat regular-sized meals, take your time and chew your food well.
* Avoid eating late at night.
* Cut down on high-fat foods if they are related to symptoms during or after eating.
* If you believe spicy foods cause symptoms, trial their restriction for a period of time. It's more likely, however, that the symptoms are related to other ingredients in a spicy curry, like FODMAPs such as onion or garlic.
* Avoid binge drinking and reduce your alcohol to well within the national recommendations. According to DrinkAware.ie, the low-risk weekly guidelines are 17 standard drinks spread out over one week for a man and 11 drinks for a woman.
* Caffeine may induce or worsen IBS symptoms. Monitor your intake, and if you think it may be related to your symptoms, reduce it.
* Avoid supplementing your diet with wheat bran. Ground linseeds (6–24g per day) can help relieve constipation, abdominal discomfort and bloating if you have constipation.
* Ensure you drink plenty of fluids (preferably water). A total of 1.5–3 litres per day is recommended.
* If you suspect that milk is a problem, you could trial a low-lactose diet to see if your symptoms improve.

Inflammatory bowel disease (IBD)

Inflammatory bowel disease includes both Crohn's disease (CD) and ulcerative colitis (UC). Both CD and UC cause inflammation in the gut. The disease can be active and inactive over time.

In CD, the inflammation can be anywhere from the mouth to the anus, although it is most common in the small intestine or colon. In UC, the inflammation is only found in the colon and rectum.

IBD can cause symptoms similar to IBS: diarrhoea, abdominal pain and bloating. In CD the inflammation can interfere with the body's ability to digest food and absorb nutrients.

People with inactive IBD may also have IBS or IBS-like symptoms, and a low FODMAP diet may be beneficial. However, it's important to note that it has not been found to be useful for people with active IBD.

Coeliac disease

Coeliac disease is an autoimmune disease. Symptoms can include any of the following: tiredness and anaemia, skin rashes, unexplained weight loss, mouth ulcers, numbness or tingling in the hands or feet and infertility.

Gut symptoms include diarrhoea and/or constipation, bloating, abdominal pain and nausea. Because these gut symptoms are so similar to IBS symptoms, it is vital to be medically diagnosed, not self-diagnosed. People may feel better when they avoid bread and pasta and be tempted to continue to exclude gluten without fully confirming a diagnosis. This can be a potential disaster.

Coeliac disease is a permanent intolerance to gluten, a protein found in wheat, rye and barley. Most people with coeliac disease can eat oats, but there is a high probability of cross-contamination with other cereals. A small number of people are sensitive to pure oats. As a result, gluten-free oats are advised for all coeliacs.

Diagnosis

Your GP can carry out a blood screening test for coeliac disease. However, false positives and false negatives can occur.

The gold standard test for coeliac disease involves an endoscopy carried out by a gastroenterologist. A biopsy from the jejunum, the middle part of the small intestine, is taken.

It is not advised to trial a gluten-free diet before your blood test or biopsy. You should include gluten in more than one meal every day for at least six weeks up to the time of the test. Gluten is found in many cereals, bread, crackers, pasta and couscous.

Treatment

Coeliac disease is a permanent, lifelong condition. The treatment is a strict gluten-free diet. Even very small amounts of gluten can be damaging. If gluten is consumed, the immune system reacts and the gut lining will be damaged again.

Excessive wind

Everyone has wind and it's normal to pass wind throughout the day. Too much wind, however, can cause pain, tummy gurgling and flatulence. Some people swallow too much air when talking or eating, resulting in excessive wind. If you gulp your food, try chewing each mouthful completely with your mouth closed.

Excessive wind may also arise if there is an imbalance in the gut microbiome. Taking a probiotic supplement for one month might help alleviate this symptom.

Eating certain foods, such as brassica vegetables, may cause wind too. Culprits include cauliflower, cabbage, broccoli and legumes like beans, peas and lentils. Drinking fizzy beverages, even carbonated water, can also cause excessive wind.

Foods, medicines and chewing gum containing the artificial sweetener sorbitol also increase wind production.

There is a possibility that wind can arise as a result of lactose intolerance. The low FODMAP diet is worth trying once your doctor has ruled out associated medical conditions related to excessive wind.

Bloated tummy

Bloating or that feeling of fullness and tightness in the abdomen can be downright uncomfortable when it happens. It's often accompanied by excessive wind and recurrent belching. It occurs due to diaphragm and abdominal muscle relaxation. It's normal for abdominal muscles to relax during meals to accommodate large volumes of food, but it seems that in the IBS patient, this muscle relaxation and sagging is excessive. The diaphragm drops and the girth grows.

 A distended tummy is one that actually increases in size. A bloated tummy is one that feels full and tight. Seventy-five per cent of IBS patients have it. These two problems usually occur together, which can be very challenging and inconvenient.

Many people are curious about whether an adapted version of the low FODMAP diet would prevent bloating in the lead-up to a once-off special occasion, even if they don't have IBS. Research is unavailable on this issue. For those preparing for a special or once-off event such as a competitive sporting event, a wedding or a model shoot, tweaking your diet to adopt some of the principles of the low FODMAP diet may well help to minimise symptoms such as constipation, diarrhoea, bloating and distention. Replacing high FODMAP foods with better options (see the swap list on pages 7–8) for a day or two prior to the big day may be worth trying, despite the lack of any solid evidence to recommend this approach.

Food hypersensitivity

'Food hypersensitivity' is an overall term for any adverse reaction to food. If the reaction involves the immune system, it's an allergy. If it doesn't, it's called food intolerance.

Food intolerance can occur hours or even days after the food is eaten. Symptoms are unpleasant and upsetting. They include tummy pain or cramp, wind, vomiting and diarrhoea.

As these symptoms are similar to IBS, some patients may be tempted to cut out certain foods and follow elimination diets. However, these are not necessary and the low FODMAP diet is the advisable intervention.

Many food intolerance tests are unreliable and worthless. They are generally expensive and don't give reliable results. You can end up eating an unbalanced diet that lacks essential nutrients. If you think you need further advice, talk to your GP about a referral to a specialist. We have included a list of the main allergens at the end of each recipe.

* A list of specialists in the Republic of Ireland is available on
  www.anaphylaxisireland.ie.
* You can also find further information on the Irish Food Allergy Network on
  www.ifan.ie.
* To find a dietitian with an interest in food allergy and intolerances,
  visit www.indi.ie.

Frequently asked questions about the low FODMAP diet

What if I'm following the low FODMAP diet but also want to lose weight?

If you would like to use the change in diet necessitated by following the low FODMAP diet alongside a weight loss programme, the following advice might be useful. Going on and off fad diets gets us nowhere in the long term. A far better idea is to reduce normal portion sizes and substitute less healthy foods for healthier ones. There's no need to make drastic, unsustainable changes. When we eat food that is better nutritionally, we may even feel less hungry for the non-nutritious stuff.

* Avoid offers in supermarkets that encourage you to buy more food than you need, even when they are on your allowed list, e.g. 'buy one get one free' offers or supersized packs.
* Measure starchy foods like rice, quinoa, rice noodles, gluten-free pasta and potatoes before you cook them. You could weigh them or always use the same cup to measure out your portion. Check whether the suggested portion on dried food packets is for the product before or after cooking.
* If you are cooking for more than one meal, get the extra food ready for storing before you start eating so that you won't go back for seconds.
* Eat slowly and enjoy the taste of your food. That way you will have time to become aware of how full you are. Aim to feel comfortably full, not stuffed. Don't be afraid to leave unwanted food on the plate.
* Where possible, control your own portions and food choices. Eat what is right for you, not because the food is allowed and available or you think it will make other people happy.

Simple tips for cutting calories in your everyday cooking

Shaving off small amounts of calories every day can really help you reach your weight loss goals. Small changes over time add up to big differences and will help you drop those stubborn extra pounds. Making a few simple swaps every day can decrease your calorie intake enough to help you lose 1–2lb per week by eating 500–1,000 fewer calories per day than normal.

Making small changes to the way you cook can cut calories without depriving yourself of the things you love to eat. Here's how.

Grill, boil, bake, poach or steam wherever possible. This avoids adding unnecessary fats to your meal, and considering that 1 tablespoon of oil is around 120 calories, this can be a massive win. If you're grilling or roasting meat, remember to put the meat on a wire rack to allow excess fat to run off.

If you do need to use oil, use spray oils. Swapping regular oils for spray versions wherever you can will make a big difference to the calorie counts of meals. Three squirts of an olive oil spray comes in at only 10 calories.

Choose boiled or baked potatoes. Avoid potatoes that have been cooked with added fat (chipped, roasted, mashed with cream) and go au naturel with the humble spud. Eat the jacket too for fibre and a sense of fullness. Try new carbohydrates, such as wild rice, red rice and quinoa.

Remove visible fat from meats before cooking. Choose lean cuts. Things like sausages and cheap burgers have a high calorie and fat content without giving you the goodness you get from a simple, pure protein source. Avoid processed fatty meats and buy the best your budget allows for better-quality ingredients and better nutrition.

Remember: just because a food is allowed, it doesn't mean it's calorie free. When using hard cheese in a dish, go for mature or strong varieties – they give you more flavour while using less of the product. Grating cheese where possible will also mean that you use less. Cheese is a good source of protein, calcium and other minerals, unlike many of the foods that are allowed in Stage 1. For example, there are many gluten-free biscuits and cakes that you could choose, but they can be high in calories and devoid of healthy nutrients. Use Stage 1 as a time to review your intake of sweet and fatty treats. It's a great time to create new habits.

Pile up on veg. Low FODMAP vegetables and salads are a great way to bulk out meals without ramping up the calorie count. Whether fresh or frozen, make sure you have plenty of veg on your plate to help you feel fuller without breaking the calorie bank.

What if I'm following the low FODMAP diet but want to gain weight?

If you need to gain weight, you have to put more eating time into your day. This may mean rescheduling other activities. Plan your meal and snack times in advance and cement them into your schedule. Avoid rushing them, no matter how busy you are.

Simple tips for planning more eating time

* Eat regularly – every two to three hours – and avoid gaps longer than three hours.
* Plan nutritious, high-calorie, low-bulk snacks, such as mixed nuts and seeds (1 handful = 200 kcals); two banana biccies (page 175) (200 kcals); some dark chocolate-covered Brazil nuts; a milkshake made with almond milk, banana, vanilla and maple syrup; a lactose-free frozen yogurt; a suitable oat-based cereal; or flapjacks.
* Eat larger meals but avoid overfilling (e.g. more gluten-free bread, an extra egg in your scramble).
* If you are finding it hard to eat enough food, add more olive oil to your salads, dinners, pan and dips. An extra tablespoon can add 120 kcals to a meal. Think about ways to include at least 2 tablespoons over the course of your day. This doesn't significantly increase the volume of food you need to eat if you have a small appetite. Add oil to mashed potatoes to increase calories without the bulk.
* Boost the calorie and nutritional content of your meals, for example by adding more chopped nuts, seeds and maple syrup into your breakfast granola recipe. You can enjoy 1 tablespoon of dried fruit (e.g. raisins, sultanas, blueberries) at one serving.
* Increase your meal frequency – eat at least three meals and three snacks daily.

Sample evening snack

Food	Calories (kcals)	Carbohydrates (g)	Protein (g)
3 oat cakes	123	18	3
60g light cream cheese, thinly spread	94	2.4	5
¼ medium avocado, mashed or finely chopped (approx. 37g)	70	0.6	0.8
90g smoked salmon, divided and placed on top of each oat cake	128	0.3	22
Total	**415**	**21.3**	**30.8**

Other ingredients to increase the calories of meals or snacks

Food	Calories (kcals)	Carbohydrates (g)	Protein (g)
Two-egg omelette for supper	163	0	10
Small matchbox size of Brie (lower in fat than Cheddar, so this portion is fine)	86	0	5
50g prawns	50	0	11
Add 1 tablespoon of olive or rapeseed oil to salad dressings, soups, stir-fries, vegetables	120	0	0
Add 30g linseeds to porridge, soups or salads	153	Trace	6.3
Add 2 tablespoons smooth peanut butter to rice cakes or toast	190	4.6	6.8
Add 2 tablespoons sesame seed spread to rice cakes or use as a dip for raw veg	199	4.3	4.2
Snack on olives, e.g. 30g snack packs available in health shops, or add to salads	53	0.3	0.4
Include oily fish such as salmon at least twice a week (per 100g steamed salmon)	200	0	21.8

What is the gut–brain connection and how does it impact IBS?

The brain and gut are closely connected and influence each other. In fact, the gut is sometimes referred to as the second brain.

It's a two-way communication route. Sensory neurons in the gut tell your brain you're satiated when your stomach is full.

Equally, how and what you think has a direct effect on the gut. Even the thought of eating helps you release digestive juices in the stomach. You can also feel butterflies in the tummy, sick to your stomach or simply nauseous as a result of your feelings and emotions.

Your gut can be distressed as a result of anxiety, stress or depression. In other words, your thoughts and emotions can affect movement and contractions in the gut, resulting in discomfort and pain. Studies have identified significantly higher stress levels in IBS patients compared with healthy subjects.

Cognitive behavioural therapy (CBT) may help improve symptoms and quality of life by helping you reframe negative thought patterns into more positive and productive ways of thinking.

 After just 12 weeks of cognitive behavioural therapy, 70 per cent of patients with IBS reported less pain, bloating and diarrhoea.

Stress-related symptoms in the gut can vary greatly from one person to the next. CBT and other relaxation treatments can help you decrease anxiety and thereby cope better with IBS.

Website and CBT resources include:

* Irish Council for Psychotherapy: www.psychotherapy-ireland.com/members/ disciplines/cognitive-behavioural-therapy/
* Institute of Cognitive Behavioural Therapy – Ireland: www.icbt.ie
* Cognitive Behavioural Psychotherapy Ireland: nacbt.ie

Explore some relaxation techniques
* Yoga or exercise of your choice
* Mindfulness meditation (see below)
* Music therapy
* Massage therapy

Mindfulness
Mindfulness (MF) offers a powerful approach to promoting emotional balance, greater resilience to stress and enjoying healthier and happier relationships.

MF is about paying attention on purpose and without judgement. It's not about getting lost in the moment – it's about waking up to the moment. It's about switching out of 'automatic pilot' mode and realising you are not your thoughts or your feelings. Some people mistakenly think that MF is a relaxation technique. It's not. It's about realisation.

MF teaches you to become an observer of your own thoughts. Thoughts are like a river. The river can be turbulent and it's easy to get swept away by stress and anxious thoughts in the heat of the moment. MF helps you to step back onto the riverbank and observe the river from a distance. You are no longer in the river, being overwhelmed by its speed and turbulence.

With repeated practice, you learn to place your awareness on something, as opposed to letting it *fall* onto something. You become conscious of where your attention is.

MF doesn't slow you down so that you can't succeed with your goals and ambitions. It keeps you in the present instead of worrying about the future or ruminating about the past.

At the start you cultivate little spots of MF throughout the day, and as you practise you begin to join up these spots into lengthier stretches of mindfulness.

Despite the fact that MF has been around for centuries, nowadays we can measure its effects. We can see the evidence that it works through functional MRI scans.

MF improves emotion regulation. Grey matter in the brain associated with depression lessens with ongoing practice. The amygdala (responsible for our fight-or-flight response) shrinks. MF techniques improve our physical as well as mental health in many ways.

According to the Harvard Health Guide, mindfulness can:

* Help relieve stress
* Alleviate gastrointestinal difficulties
* Treat heart disease
* Lower blood pressure
* Reduce chronic pain
* Improve sleep

You can begin with either of two evidenced-based eight-week courses: mindfulness-based stress reduction or mindfulness-based cognitive therapy.

Should I take probiotics when following the low FODMAP diet, and if so, when?

Bacteria are natural gut residents. Some are good, some not so good. Certain bacteria help to break down food and produce gas as a by-product of digestion. Too much of the wrong type of bacteria can result in poor digestion, bloating and excessive gas. Gut bacteria in IBS patients seems to differ from the microbiome of healthy people. Research suggests that low doses of friendly bacteria or probiotics may improve certain symptoms by tipping the balance in favour of the good bacteria. Unfortunately, not everyone responds to probiotic therapy. Currently there is no means of assessing an individual's microbiome and no way of knowing whether a probiotic supplement would be of benefit or not.

However, if your symptoms are severe, it's worth trying a probiotic supplement for a minimum of four weeks either before or after the low FODMAP diet. That way you can be sure that any improvement is attributable to the probiotic supplement as opposed to the low FODMAP diet.

The majority of people who respond can expect a reduction of symptoms, not a complete eradication of symptoms. The benefits are also very specific to the probiotic strain used.

With so many probiotic supplements with variable strains and doses of bacteria, it can be difficult to know what's best to take. In order for the probiotic to work it must 'arrive, survive and thrive' where it's needed. For this reason, it's important to discuss your symptoms with your dietitian. There are certain probiotic supplements that specifically impact on bloating and constipation but might have little effect on loose stools. Some probiotics require a prescription.

The following probiotics have published research to support their use for specific gut symptoms:

* **Alflorex (B. infantis 35624):** Reduces bloating, cramping and stool frequency.
* **Liquid Symprove:** Improvement in overall IBS symptom severity.
* **Powdered VSL-3:** Improvement in bloating in diarrhoea dominant IBS.

Note: If you find a particular probiotic beneficial, you can continue taking it, but the long-term effects are not known yet.

How our food choices affect the microbiome

It seems that a diet rich in nutritious foods is associated with a greater diversity of bacteria living in the gut. On the flip side, less nutritious diets are associated with poor diversity, reduced gut functionality and fewer health benefits.

The natural balance of gut bacteria is altered by our dietary choices (not just by probiotic supplements). As a result, researchers are striving to understand the effects of the low FODMAP diet on gut bacteria. Many natural prebiotic foods (such as beans and lentils) are restricted in portion size temporarily and sometimes for the longer term if they are trigger foods. What implications this may have is as yet unknown.

Other IBS aids

* **Peppermint oil** can slow the time it takes food to travel through the gut and lessen diarrhoea in some people.
* Less than 2 tablespoons (50g) of **probiotic yogurt** is allowed in the first stage of the low FODMAP diet. The same rule applies to kefir, an alternative source of these friendly bacteria. Check with your dietitian or your FODMAP app for suitable brands if you want to include some kefir in your diet.

✳ Making a water-based **kefir** allows you to enjoy more of this affordable fermented food. It's simply a matter of adding kefir grains to sweetened water in a big glass jar and leaving it, covered, at room temperature for one or more days. The culture works its magic and you can get the consistency you desire with a little trial and error. Numerous health claims are made about kefir, but additional and larger studies are needed before any can be verified. You can buy the grains online and there are numerous YouTube videos explaining how to make it. You can flavour kefir with vanilla, but not honey.

 Prebiotic foods encourage the growth of friendly bacteria. However, prebiotics can worsen IBS symptoms in some people. Many are eliminated during Stage 1 of the low FODMAP diet. If you wish to take a probiotic supplement, make sure it is prebiotic free, as sometimes they are found together in supplements.

Excluded prebiotics during Stage 1

✳ Chicory root and inulin	✳ Garlic
✳ Onions	✳ Fennel bulb
✳ Globe and Jerusalem artichokes	✳ Leeks
✳ Mangetout	✳ Mushrooms
✳ Savoy cabbage	✳ Asparagus
✳ Beetroot	✳ Brussels sprouts
✳ Apricots	✳ Dried figs
✳ Grapefruit	✳ Nectarines
✳ Peaches	✳ Plums or prunes
✳ Pomegranates	✳ Watermelon
✳ Wheat	✳ Barley
✳ Rye	✳ Amaranth

Once Stage 2 (the reintroduction stage) has been completed, it is recommended to include as many of the above foods as you can tolerate in your diet in the long term. Although more research is necessary, there is a strong feeling that the long-term avoidance of these foods may have negative health consequences, as it may mess with your microbiome.

What is a safe intake of caffeine on the low FODMAP diet and what are the allowed sources?

A caffeine intake up to 400mg per day is a safe intake for the general population (except during pregnancy, when 200mg per day is the current maximum). If you are slight, please note that nervousness, anxiety and irritability have been observed with caffeine intakes of 5mg per kg of body weight per day.

Product	Serving size (unless otherwise stated)		Milligrams of caffeine (approximate values)
	oz	ml	
Coffee			
Brewed	8	237 (1 cup)	135
Roasted and ground, percolated	8	237	118
Roasted and ground, filter drip	8	237	179
Roasted and ground, decaffeinated	8	237	3
Instant	8	237	76–106
Instant decaffeinated	8	237	5
Tea			
Average blend	8	237	43
Green	8	237	30
Instant	8	237	15
Leaf or bag	8	237	50
Decaffeinated tea	8	237	0
Cola beverages			
Cola beverage, regular	12	355 (1 can)	36–46
Cola beverage, diet	12	355	39–50

Note: Values in the table were referenced from the following sources: Harland, B.F. (2000), 'Caffeine and nutrition', Nutrition, 16(7–8):522–526. Shils, et al. (1999), Modern nutrition in health and disease, 9th edition, Williams & Wilkins, Waverly Company, Baltimore.

What should I do about fibre intake while on the diet?

Increasing or decreasing your fibre intake can help IBS symptoms. The amount of fibre you need will vary depending on your symptoms, your tolerance of high-fibre foods and your current fibre intake.

* If you already include a lot of high-fibre foods and have uncontrolled symptoms such as diarrhoea, distention and bloating, consider reducing your intake of fibre to see if your symptoms improve.
* If you feel you don't eat enough fibre, consider increasing your intake gradually. It's important to introduce each new fibre food every one to two days to let your bowel adapt to the extra fibre. Also, make sure you take more fluids with added fibre.

There are two main types of fibre:

* **Insoluble fibre** or 'roughage', which is found in foods such as brown and wild rice, skins of potatoes, fruit and vegetables, and nuts and seeds.
* **Soluble fibre** is found in oats, fruit and vegetables, peas, beans, lentils, nuts and seeds.

You may also want to refer to the table below for additional changes you can make to your diet.

CONSTIPATION	DIARRHOEA	WIND AND BLOATING
* Try increasing your fibre intake from allowed foods during Stage 1.	* If you eat high-fibre foods, reduce your fibre intake from the allowed foods in Stage 1. Stick to rice crackers and corncakes without added fibre and white wheat-free and gluten-free bread and rolls.	* Reduce insoluble fibre (e.g. fruit and vegetable skins) but include more soluble fibre (oats and linseeds) during Stage 1.
* Use wholegrain varieties of rice, buckwheat and oat breads and cereals and ensure you drink plenty of water, as this helps work with the fibre to ease constipation.	* If symptoms improve, you can increase your fibre intake again to assess your tolerance level of these foods.	* If this makes a clear difference to your symptoms, you can gradually reintroduce these skins until you find your tolerance level again.
* Do not use wheat bran supplements, as they may make symptoms worse. Try oat bran instead.	* Avoid sorbitol (an artificial sweetener found in sugar-free or 'diet' sweets, gum, drinks and in some diabetic and slimming products).	* Include a maximum of three portions of fruit per day, spread out throughout the day. Limit juice to one small glass per day.
* Try adding ground or whole linseeds to cereal, salad or 2 tablespoons of natural yogurt. Start with 1 teaspoon, increasing to 1 tablespoon per day over time and as tolerated. Drink 150ml additional water with each tablespoon. It may take up to three months to notice an effect.		* If you find alcohol makes symptoms worse, cut down on your alcohol intake.

Symptom assessment for IBS

1 Do you currently have satisfactory relief of your gut symptoms?
(Tick one.)

☐ Yes   ☐ No

**2 Rate your symptoms during the last two weeks by placing
a tick in the box that best describes each symptom.**
(Tick 'none' if you do not have this symptom.)

	NONE (no symptoms or very rarely)	MILD (occasional or mild symptoms)	MODERATE (frequent symptoms that affect some social activities)	SEVERE (continuous symptoms that affect most social activities)
Abdominal pain/discomfort				
Abdominal bloating/distention				
Increased flatulence/wind				
Belching or burping				
Stomach/abdominal gurgling				
Urgency to open bowels				
Incomplete evacuation (inability to pass all stool)				
Nausea				
Heartburn				
Acid regurgitation				
Tiredness/lethargy				
Overall symptoms				

3 **Currently, how often do you pass a bowel action?**
(Tick one box.)

☐ Once a week

☐ Once every four to six days

☐ Once every two to three days

☐ Once a day

☐ Two to three times a day

☐ Four to six times a day

☐ Seven or more times a day

4 **If relevant, how many weeks did it take for your symptoms to improve on the low FODMAP diet?**

[   ] weeks ☐ N/A

Index

T